Herbal
HOME SPA

A Natural Approach to Beautiful
Hair, Skin, Hands, and Feet

Stephanie L. Tourles ❧ Norma Pasekoff Weinberg

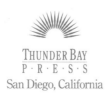

THUNDER BAY
P · R · E · S · S
San Diego, California

Thunder Bay Press
An imprint of the Advantage Publishers Group
5880 Oberlin Drive, San Diego, CA 92121-4794
www.advantagebooksonline.com

Edited by Deborah Balmuth and Karen Levy
Original text design by Carol J. Jessop, Black Trout Design
Text production by Susan Bernier and Kelley Nesbit
Indexed by Eileen M. Clawson

This book has been excerpted from *The Herbal Body Book* (Storey, 1994), *Natural Hand Care* (Storey, 1998), *Natural Foot Care* (Storey, 1998), and *Naturally Healthy Skin* (Storey, 1999).

All notations of errors or omissions should be addressed to Thunder Bay Press, editorial department, at the above address. All other correspondence (author inquiries, permissions) concerning the content of this book should be addressed to Storey Publishing, 210 MASS MoCA Way, North Adams, MA 01247.

ISBN 1-57145-812-3
Library of Congress Cataloging-in-Publication Data available upon request.

Printed in the United States by R.R. Donnelley
10 9 8 7 6 5 4 3 2 1

TABLE OF CONTENTS

For my husband, Bill, who is always there

with his constant love, support, strong self-discipline,

and drive to succeed. To my parents, Mike and Brenda Anchors,

for their guidance and patience, and for instilling in me

courage to pursue my lifelong dreams. And to my grandparents,

Earl and Phenie Ashe and Grace and the late Jack Anchors.

— *Stephanie L. Tourles*

I want to thank everyone who lent me a hand in this project: the reference

libraries in Cape Cod and Boston public libraries; the Herb Society of America;

the herbalists and other experts interviewed, who freely shared their time,

energy, and wisdom; and the reviewers, Robert Folety, Ila Hirsch, Michael Janson,

M.D., Larry B. Meyerson, M.D., Lawrence A. Norton, M.D.,

and Nikolaus J. Smeh, for their patient advice.

— *Norma Pasekoff Weinberg*

INTRODUCTION

One of the greatest treasures that a woman or a man can have is healthy, radiant skin. A beautiful complexion and glorious skin are a reflection of our personal life-style practices. The most rigorously followed healthful living plan necessarily includes a nutritious diet, pure water, regular exercise in the fresh air, adequate rest and sleep, sensible stress management, and an effective skin cleansing program. It is this last part, effective skin cleansing, with which this book is intimately concerned.

I am a licensed aesthetician in the Commonwealth of Massachusetts. My specialty is helping individuals achieve their rightful heritage as a "beautiful person," as well as helping them claim their highest health potential through natural procedures.

In my years of experience, I have worked with many commercially prepared products from first-class department stores, as well as with many so-called "natural" products from health food stores. Many of these skin and body cleansers and moisturizers contain highly toxic and irritating ingredients. I have frequently had clients come to me suffering from allergic reactions to these often costly products. Their suffering led me to experiment with totally natural, totally wholesome cosmetic ingredients. My success with this experimentation led to the writing of this book.

By preparing my own facial and body cleansers from fresh herbs, grains, fruits, vegetables, nuts, seeds, and oils, right in my very own kitchen, I have created recipes that produce the desired result of virtually all commercial cosmetics. And with the help and instructions in this book, you too can create natural, health-loving cosmetics that bring a radiance and glow to your face and whole body.

As you're probably aware, commercial cosmetics have one of the highest profit markups of any product on the market. The cost to produce the bottle, label it, and package it is often more than the few cents worth of ingredients in the bottle. In fact, it is not uncommon to pay $20 or more for a two-ounce (60-ml) jar of cream that promises to rejuvenate you by twenty years in twenty days! We all know such a promise can never be kept, but we pay the price anyway because the promise feels so good.

Aside from the obvious savings, creating your own cosmetics at home has many other advantages:

◆ You have a choice of the purest, freshest, most natural ingredients available. Many of these you probably have in your kitchen cupboard or refrigerator, or can easily purchase them from local health food stores, specialty shops, or mail-order herb companies.

◆ You can customize natural cosmetics to match your particular skin type or hair condition.

◆ You can scent your cosmetics with your favorite herbal fragrance.

◆ By creating your own personal care products, you are contributing to keeping the earth green. Homemade cosmetics contain no toxic chemicals to pollute the earth, they require no animal testing, and the packaging can be recycled.

◆ In short, nature has truly rewarded us with a multitude of all-natural, wholesome ingredients with which to create a variety of products to both cleanse and nourish your skin, hair, nails, and more.

On the following pages are simple directions for making facial, hair, and body cleansers. You will find chapters offering facial steams, masks, creams, lotions, toners, and hair products, to use and give as gifts. You'll also find a listing of where to buy any unfamiliar ingredients, specifically herbs. In the spirit of realism and economy, beauty and health, I wish you well!

REMEMBER: Nature's Promise . . .
Take care of your skin
and your skin will reward you with
health and beauty for the rest of your life.

—Stephanie L. Tourles

PART I:
HERBAL BODY TREATMENTS

A Natural Approach
to Healthier Skin and Hair

Stephanie L. Tourles

CHAPTER 1

A Natural Approach to Beautiful Skin

▼▼▼▼

In order to properly care for your skin, it's important that you understand something about its structure and purpose. With this understanding, you'll be better prepared to make decisions about how and why to care for your skin.

The word "system," according to the *Random House Dictionary,* can be defined as a group or combination of things or parts forming a complex or unified whole. Your skin is a *living system.* Just one square inch consists of approximately 19 million cells, 625 sweat glands, 94 sebaceous glands, 60 hairs, 19,000 sensory nerve cells, 1,250 pain receptors, 13 cold and 78 heat receptors, 160 pressure receptors, and 19 yards of blood vessels.

Your skin serves the body in many capacities, including:

♦ sensory perception
♦ protecting underlying tissues from injury and dehydration
♦ assisting in processes of temperature maintenance and toxic waste elimination
♦ serving as the origination point for the manufacture of vitamin D
♦ giving structure to all organs and systems within the body

To say the least, your skin is an integral part of your living being and one that plays a vital role within your body's supportive and functional capacities. It's essential that you learn how to care for it and nourish it so that it will remain healthy regardless of the climate you live in or your chronological age.

Contrary to popular opinion, beautiful skin doesn't come in pretty bottles filled with a vitamin/hormone cream that smells of artificial fragrance. Nor does it come from chemicals designed to dry up acne pimples, such as tetracycline, Accutane, or benzoyl peroxide. Truly beautiful skin comes as a result of adhering to a program of feeding your body a proper diet, getting daily exercise and adequate sleep, and by employing an appropriate cleansing regime.

Though this book is primarily concerned with natural skin care through the use of wholesome products, I want to stress the importance of a proper diet and daily exercise in maintaining beautiful skin.

DIET

The skin is one of the first organs of the body to be affected by poor diet, vitamin and mineral deficiencies, and improper elimination. Moist, clear, radiant skin is generally a sign of good health, while skin that is dry and flaky or oily and pimply can be indicative of internal problems, especially where nutrition is concerned.

Your diet should consist of foods that are high in complex carbohydrates, low in fat, high in fiber, and moderate in protein. A wide variety of foods in their whole, natural state should be consumed daily, including several servings each of fresh and dried fruits, vegetables, whole grains, plus a few fresh nuts and seeds. If you consume dairy products, they should be non-fat, and cheeses should be eaten in moderation because of their high fat content. Meat eaters should try to limit their meat consumption to three to four ounces (85 to 133 g) per day (about the size of a deck of cards) and try to buy only free-range chickens; fresh, deep-sea fish; and extremely lean beef that was raised without hormones and antibiotics. Of course, it goes without saying, one should eliminate smoking and consume alcohol in small amounts, if at all.

A wholesome, balanced diet such as this nourishes the inner body and is reflected on the outer body as gorgeous skin. As you plan your daily or weekly menus, try to remember that your skin is the visible evidence of the condition of your inner health. It is the mirror that reflects your present state of health or ill-health.

EXERCISE

Daily exercise is vital to your physical well-being, and can help your mental health as well by eliminating or reducing stress. By taking a brisk 30-minute walk and performing approximately 15 minutes of gentle stretches each and every day, you stimulate your metabolism, keep your muscles and joints loose and flexible, enjoy a bit of fresh air and sunshine, and get your heart pumping and blood flowing. Try to exercise vigorously enough so that you work up a good sweat. Sweating cools your skin and eliminates waste through your pores.

If you don't like to walk, choose whatever you enjoy: biking, jogging, swimming, aerobic classes, tennis, or even roller blading. There really is something for everyone. It's up to you to find it and stick with it.

If you are over the age of thirty-five, have been inactive for a period of time, or have any health problems, be sure to get your doctor's okay *before* beginning any exercise program. For further information on diet and exercise, see the Resources for reading suggestions.

CARING FOR YOUR SKIN

To keep your skin deep-down clean, no matter whether it's oily, combination, normal, or dry, all that is necessary is that you observe these five basic practices: cleansing, toning (sometimes referred to as clarifying or freshening), moisturizing, high water intake, and dry brushing. The first three should be performed as a series of steps. Here's how:

1. Cleansing: This step, I feel, is the most important. Twice a day, using a washcloth or facial sponge, apply the appropriate facial cleanser for your skin type to your face and throat and massage gently, using upward, circular strokes. This step should take about a minute. Now, rinse your face with clean, warm water to remove all traces of the cleanser and pat dry.

Never, never, never *scrub* your facial skin! I've actually seen some women scrub their face so hard you'd think they were trying to clean their kitchen sink! Always be gentle. Now, on to the next step.

2. Toning: A toner or astringent is designed to remove any traces of cleanser that have been left behind during the cleansing process and to restore the skin to its normally acid pH. To apply your toner, simply saturate a 100% cotton ball with your chosen herbal liquid and apply to your face and throat using gentle, upward strokes. Do not pat dry. You want to lock in this precious moisture by performing the next step.

3. Moisturizing: Using a moisturizer should become a part of everyone's daily routine regardless of whether you think your skin is too oily to benefit from one or not. A moisturizer is designed to prevent dehydration (loss of water) from occurring in your skin. Your skin can be extremely oily, but also suffer from a lack of water. A good moisturizer serves as a barrier between your skin and the environment. It will help to keep your skin younger-looking longer.

To benefit from all that a moisturizer has to offer, simply apply the appropriate moisturizer to your already moist face and throat, using upward, circular strokes until the moisturizer disappears. You're finished!

These three steps should take you no longer than five minutes, twice a day — a small amount of time to devote daily for a lifetime of beautiful skin!

Finally, let me mention the two last secrets for beautiful skin: drinking pure, clean water and dry brushing.

TAKING THE MYSTERY OUT OF pH

You've seen it on everything from shampoos to soap, but what exactly is pH? The pH (potential hydrogen) of a liquid refers to its degree of acidity or alkalinity. Meters and indicator papers have been developed for the measurement of pH. The pH scale goes from 0 to 14, with the neutral point being 7. Anything below a 7 on the pH scale is regarded as acid. The lower the pH, the greater the degree of acidity. Anything above a 7 is regarded as alkaline. The higher the pH, the greater is the degree of alkalinity. The pH of normal, healthy skin ranges from 4.5 to 6 and is most often referred to as 5.5. Your skin maintains its proper pH level by forming an acid mantle on its surface from the combined secretions of your sweat and oil glands. By using a toner to keep your skin at its proper pH level, you help prevent bacterial penetration (which occurs when skin is too acidic) and flaking and scaling because of moisture loss (which occurs when skin is too alkaline).

Regardless of your skin type, you should always look for a toner with a pH level in the range of 4.5 to 6.

4. Drink plenty of water: Whether in the form of raw fruits and vegetables or several glasses of plain water, sufficient water consumption is essential to maintaining soft, moist, glowing skin. Any model will tell you that he or she drinks a minimum of six glasses a day. I personally enjoy four to six glasses, plus consuming a high water content diet.

For those of you who just hate plain water, try adding a squeeze of lime, lemon, or orange juice. This will turn your plain, blah water into a very refreshing drink. A splash of cranberry juice tastes great too!

5. Dry brushing: Dry brushing is a must for smooth, clear skin. Over the course of a day your skin eliminates more than a pound of waste through thousands of tiny sweat glands. In fact, about one-third of all the body's impurities are excreted this way. But, if your pores are clogged by tight-fitting clothes, aluminum-containing antiperspirants, and mineral oil-based moisturizers, there's no way for these toxic by-products to escape. Over time, your skin will begin to look pale, pasty, and pimply.

> ### A DRY BRUSH BONUS
> Here's an added plus to dry brushing . . . because dry-brushing opens your clogged pores and aids in elimination, your cellulite will begin to diminish. Trust me . . . it works. Follow a good, low-fat diet and exercise program, and it will work even faster.

Dry brushing is performed on dry skin — not oiled, not damp, but dry before you shower. Using a natural-fiber brush the size of your palm, preferably with a handle, you simply brush your entire body — except your face (and breasts, if you're a woman) — for 5 to 10 minutes. Daily. Do not brush hard. You will have to start very gently and work your way up to more vigorous brushing, but never scrub. It will take your skin a while to get used to this new treatment. Begin brushing your hands first, in between the fingers, then arms, underarms, neck, chest, stomach, back, then on to each leg beginning with the feet. You will feel wonderfully invigorated when finished, and your skin will glow! Then, just jump in the shower, and all of the dead skin you just exfoliated is washed away. Be sure to pat, not rub, your skin dry, and apply a light moisturizer after you shower.

Wash your brush with soap and water every week or so to keep it free of skin debris.

SUN EXPOSURE

Light to moderate exposure to the sun makes us feel good, it helps the body manufacture vitamin D, gives us energy after a long, cold winter, it warms the soul, and leaves a rosy-golden glow upon the skin. On the flipside, overexposure dries our skin, causes wrinkles, blotchiness, and premature aging, and increasingly, leads to skin cancer.

In my opinion, 10 to 20 minutes of sun exposure each day, (without sunscreen), *before* 10:30 a.m. or *after* 4:30 p.m., is good for your physical health as well as your emotional well-being. There are many that disagree with me, but I feel that with such a light exposure to the sun, the benefits outweigh any possible harm.

However, if you are going to be in the sun for a longer period of time, by all means apply a good sunscreen. This is especially important if you're going to be on or near water, or even relaxing on a sandy beach. Water and sand can reflect the sun's powerful rays, further increasing the chances of overexposure and skin damage. I always wear a sunscreen with a sun protection factor (SPF) of at least 15. You may need an even stronger one, depending on your skin type.

If you want to preserve the beauty of your skin for years to come and help prevent skin cancer, do not spend excess time in the sun, unprotected.

GIFT IDEA

Know any sun worshippers? Everyone does! By March 1, they're outside trying to get a jump on their summer tan, even if there's still snow on the ground! Many of these people aren't too keen on using sunscreen, either, but I'm sure they would appreciate a bottle of your freshly made, low SPF Sunscreen Body Oil (see page 72).

Fill an 8-ounce (240 ml) plastic squeeze bottle with your wonderful-smelling creation, apply a decorative label, and tie a piece of twine with a couple of seashells attached to each end, around the top.

CHAPTER 2
All-Natural Cosmetic Recipes

The sections that follow contain recipes for making natural products for the face, body, hair, and more. The ingredients are easy to find and the recipes are relatively simple to make.

All herbs used in the following recipes are dried unless otherwise specified. If you have access to fresh herbs, then you may want to dry the herbs yourself. Recently dried herbs have a wonderful, just-picked aroma and will make your products all the more delightful.

A "recipe key," to the right of each ingredient list, gives a quick summary as well as some added tips. Use to tell whether that particular cosmetic is right for your skin or hair type.

MAKING MEAL BLENDS

Three main ingredients you'll always want to have on hand are almond meal, ground oatmeal, and sunflower seed meal.

Almond Meal

To make one-half cup (125 ml) of *almond meal,* blend approximately 50 large, raw almonds in the blender or food processor until the consistency is like finely grated parmesan cheese.

Ground Oatmeal

To make one-half cup (125 ml) of *ground oatmeal,* blend one cup of old-fashioned oats in the blender or food processor until it feels like fine flour.

Sunflower Seed Meal

To make one-half cup (125 ml) of *sunflower seed meal,* grind ¾ cup (180 ml) of large seeds (hulled), until the consistency is also like parmesan cheese.

HERBS AND INGREDIENTS THAT MAY CAUSE IRRITATION TO EYES AND SKIN

Almond, bitter, essential oil

Aloe Vera, skin of fresh leaf and gel

Benzoin, tincture of

Chamomile

Cinnamon, essential oil

Clove, essential oil

Cocoa Butter

Cornstarch

Glycerin

Lanolin

Lemon, essential oil

Lemongrass, essential oil

Lime, essential oil

Orange, essential oil

Synthetic essential oils

Tangerine, essential oil

Vinegar

A FEW WORDS ABOUT SAFETY

Many of these recipes look and smell edible because the majority of ingredients are edible. This does not mean that these products are safe to consume, though. Please, for safety's (and your tastebuds') sake, clearly label all products and keep away from children.

If you are allergy prone, test yourself for adverse reactions to the herbs called for in the recipe. To do this, try a patch test. Prepare a paste with 1 teaspoon (5 ml) of the herb in question and a small amount of boiling water. Apply the paste to cleaned skin on the inside of your elbow. Cover with an adhesive bandage and leave on for 24 hours. To test an essential oil, dilute one drop with one tablespoon of water, saturate a cotton ball, and apply the same way as the paste. If a rash or redness appears, do not use the herb (or oil). Substitute with another that causes no reaction.

If anything enters your eyes and an irritation develops, promptly flood your eyes with cool water repeatedly. If the irritation continues, see a doctor immediately.

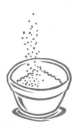

FACIAL AND BODY SCRUBS

A cosmetic scrub is used to remove dry, dead skin cells from the surface of the skin. It can be used on all skin types except those with severe acne, thread (spider) veins, or highly sensitive skin. A scrub may be too irritating for these conditions. These recipes should be used on facial and body areas only, unless otherwise specified.

Please note: When using any of these exfoliants, do not "scrub" your face and neck. Your body may be able to tolerate a bit more friction, but your delicate facial and neck skin cannot. Please allow the product to do the work for you and be very gentle.

For the face: Using a light touch with your fingers or a facial cloth, massage your face and neck in a circular, upward motion. Do this for approximately 1 minute. Rinse thoroughly. Avoid eye area at all times!

For the body: Scrubs may be applied to your body simply by using your hands or you may wish to use a body loofah, washcloth, or body brush. Use whatever feels best to you. I prefer to use the body scrubs in the shower, as they tend to be a bit messy.

GIFT IDEA

Facial and body scrubs make great gifts for men or women. Make up a cup or two of the scrub that best suits the recipient's skin type, put it in a regular plastic food storage bag, tie with a ribbon or twine, and place in a decorative tin, box, or gift bag with a nice note. Make sure you include complete instructions with your gift.

ALL-PURPOSE SCRUB

½ cup (125 ml) ground
  oatmeal
⅓ cup (80 ml) ground
   sunflower seeds
4 tablespoons (60 ml)
  almond meal
½ teaspoon (2.5 ml)
  ground peppermint,
  spearmint, or rosemary
  leaves
dash cinnamon powder
  (optional)
water, milk, or heavy cream

Good for: all skin types
Use: daily or as needed
Follow with: moisturizer
Prep time: approximately 10 minutes
Mix with: blender, food processor
Store in: zip-seal bag, low tub/jar, or tin
Yields: 4 to 24 treatments,
depending on use
Special: Leaves skin
very smooth.

Mix dry ingredients together thoroughly. Use approximately 2 teaspoons (10 ml) of scrub mixture for the face, more for the body, and enough water (for oily skin), milk (for normal skin), or heavy cream (for dry skin), to form a spreadable paste. Allow to thicken for 1 minute. Massage onto face and throat or body area. Rinse.

GENTLE FACIAL EXFOLIANT

2 tablespoons (30 ml)
  powdered milk
½ cup (125 ml) ground
  oatmeal
1 teaspoon (5 ml) cornmeal
water

Good for: all skin types, especially dry
and sensitive
Use: daily or as needed
Follow with: moisturizer
Prep time: approximately 5 minutes
Mix with: small bowl and spoon
Store in: zip-seal bag, low tub/jar, or tin
Yields: approximately 10 treatments
Special: Leaves skin silky soft.

Mix dry ingredients thoroughly. Combine 1 tablespoon (15 ml) of scrub mixture with enough water to form a spreadable paste. Allow to thicken for 1 minute. Massage onto face and throat. Rinse.

SCRUB FOR OILY SKIN

½ cup (125 ml) ground
oatmeal
½ cup (125 ml) almond
meal
1 tablespoon (15 ml) sea
salt
1 teaspoon (5 ml) ground
peppermint leaves
1 teaspoon (5 ml) ground
rosemary leaves
astringent of choice (see
recipes on pages 24–29)

Good for: normal and oily skin
Use: three times per week
Follow with: astringent, then moisturizer
Prep time: approximately 10 minutes
Mix with: blender or food processor
Store in: zip-seal bag, low tub/jar, or tin
Yields: approximately 16 treatments
Special: Great for oily areas on shoulders, chest, and back.

Throughly mix all dry ingredients. Mix 1 tablespoon (15 ml) of scrub with enough astringent to form a paste. Allow to thicken. Massage gently onto face and throat. Rinse.

BODY SCRUB

¼ cup (60 ml) sea salt
¼ cup (60 ml) warmed
coconut or olive oil

Good for: all skin types
Use: as desired
Follow with: moisturizer, if desired
Prep time: approximately 5 minutes
Mix with: small bowl and spoon
Store in: Make recipe only as needed.
Do not store.
Yields: 1 treatment
Special: Leaves calloused areas especially soft.

Stir both ingredients together. Massage onto body with hands or mitt using a light, but firm, pressure. Continue massaging, not rubbing, until a rosy glow appears. Rinse with warm water, towel dry.

CREAMY SCRUB CLEANSER

2 tablespoons (30 ml)
  heavy cream (or 1 tablespoon [15 ml] cream
  and 1 tablespoon [15 ml]
  peach pureé)
1 tablespoon (15 ml)
  ground oatmeal
1 teaspoon (5 ml)
  sunflower seed meal
½ teaspoon (2.5 ml)
  chamomile flowers

Good for: normal and dry skin
Use: daily or as desired
Follow with: moisturizer
Prep time: 5 to 10 minutes
Mix with: mortar and pestle or small bowl and fork
Store in: Dry mix: zip-seal bag, low tub/jar, or tin
Yields: 1 treatment
Special: May use as mask — allow to dry 15 to 20 minutes. Rinse. Very soothing.

Mix ingredients together to form a very creamy paste. Massage onto face and throat. Allow mixture to remain on your face for approximately 5 minutes. Rinse. Used frequently, your skin should acquire a "peaches and cream" glow!

ALMOND MEAL CLEANSER

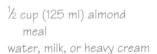

½ cup (125 ml) almond
  meal
water, milk, or heavy cream

Good for: all skin types
Use: daily or as desired
Follow with: moisturizer
Prep time: approximately 5 minutes
Mix with: small bowl and spoon
Store in: Dry mix: zip-seal bag, low tub/jar, or tin
Yields: approximately 12 treatments

Mix 2 teaspoons (10 ml) of almond meal with enough liquid to form a paste. Spread onto moistened face and throat and gently massage for 1 minute. Rinse with warm water.

OATMEAL SMOOTHER

½ cup (125 ml) ground
   oatmeal
½ cup (125 ml) powdered
   milk
water

Good for: all skin types, especially dry,
delicate, sensitive skin

Use: daily or as desired

Follow with: moisturizer

Prep time: approximately 5 minutes

Mix with: small bowl and spoon

Store in: Dry mix: zip-seal bag, low
tub/jar, or tin

Yields: approximately 24 treatments

Special: Leaves skin very smooth and soft.

Mix 2 teaspoons (10 ml) of scrub mixture with 2 teaspoons (10 ml) water.
Stir until a smooth paste forms. Massage onto face and throat. Rinse.

BALANCING SCRUB

1 tablespoon (15 ml)
   papaya pulp or plain
   yogurt
2 teaspoons (10 ml)
   ground oatmeal
1 teaspoon (5 ml) sea salt

Good for: oily and normal-to-dry skin

Use: two times per week

Follow with: moisturizer

Prep time: approximately 5 minutes

Mix with: small bowl and fork

Store in: Make recipe only as needed.
Do not store.

Yields: 1 treatment

Special: Good for blotchy or unevenly colored skin.

Combine ingredients and massage mixture onto face and throat until a
rosy glow appears. Leave on for 5 minutes. Rinse with cool water. Use this
scrub every week until your skin begins to become more uniformly colored and has attained a smooth appearance.

SENSATIONAL SUNFLOWER FRICTION

1 tablespoon (15 ml)
   sunflower seed meal
1 tablespoon (15 ml)
   applesauce

Good for: normal and dry skin
Use: three times per week
Follow with: moisturizer
Prep time: approximately 5 minutes
Mix with: small bowl and spoon
Store in: Do not store. Mix only as needed.
Yields: 1 treatment
Special: Very moisturizing.

Combine ingredients to form a paste. Massage onto face and throat. Allow to remain for 10 minutes so that the oils of the sunflower seeds may be released and absorbed into your thirsty skin. Rinse with warm water.

PINEAPPLE/SUNFLOWER SCRUB

1 tablespoon (15 ml) sun-
   flower seed meal
1 tablespoon (15 ml) fresh
   pineapple or lemon juice
   (diluted 50% with
   water)

Good for: oily and normal-to-dry skin
Use: two times per week
Follow with: moisturizer
Prep time: 5 to 10 minutes
Mix with: small bowl and spoon
Store in: Do not store. Mix only as needed.
Yields: 1 treatment
Special: Excellent for a fading tan. Evens skin tone.

Mix ingredients thoroughly and massage onto face and throat. Include the chest area if skin tone is uneven there. Allow to dry for 10 minutes. Rinse with cool water. This scrub tends to bleach the skin slightly. Use every week until your skin takes on a smooth, even appearance.

CORNMEAL AND HONEY SCRUB

1½ teaspoons (7.5 ml)
cornmeal
½ teaspoon (2.5 ml) water
1 teaspoon (5 ml) honey

Good for: all skin types, except sensitive

Use: three times per week

Follow with: moisturizer

Prep time: approximately 5 minutes

Mix with: small bowl and spoon

Store in: Do not store. Mix only as needed.

Yields: 1 treatment

Combine ingredients thoroughly and allow to thicken for 1 minute. Massage onto face and throat and leave on for 15 minutes. Rinse with warm water.

BREWER'S YEAST AND OATMEAL SCRUB

¼ cup (60 ml) brewer's
  yeast (not baking
  yeast)
¼ cup (60 ml) ground
  oatmeal
water

Good for: oily and normal-to-dry skin
Use: two times per week
Follow with: moisturizer
Prep time: approximately 5 minutes
Mix with: small bowl and spoon
Store in: Dry mix: zip-seal bag, low
tub/jar, or tin
Yields: approximately 8 treatments
Special: Revs up the circulation — great
for a pale complexion!

Mix dry ingredients completely. Using 1 tablespoon (15 ml) scrub and approximately 1 tablespoon (15 ml) water, form a spreadable paste. Allow to thicken for 1 minute. Massage onto face and throat and allow to dry for 15 minutes. Rinse with cool water.

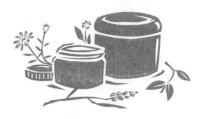

CLEANSING CREAMS AND LOTIONS

Cleansing creams and lotions are used to remove makeup and everyday dirt and grime that collects in your facial pores. Unlike using soap to cleanse your face, which has a tendency to dry the skin's surface, these products are very gentle and nourishing and do a thorough job of cleansing.

Application tip: First, moisten your face and throat with a warm, moist washcloth or several splashes of warm water. Next, apply a small amount of cleanser (about a teaspoon or two [5 to 10 ml] will do) using the pads of your fingers, with upward, circular strokes. Continue applying cleanser until your entire facial area is covered. Now, gently remove cleanser with a moistened washcloth, then splash your face several times with clean, warm water. Pat dry. You are now ready to apply the appropriate toner or astringent for your skin type.

Important "cooking" instructions: Many of the following recipes require the heating of various oils, waxes, and other ingredients so that they may be properly blended. When "cooking" your cleansing creams and lotions, please use the "low" setting on your stove to warm or melt your ingredients or use a double boiler. Never let the herbal liquid or wax/oil mixture get hot. *Warm them just enough* for the waxes to melt and the

GIFT IDEA

Freshly made cleansing creams, along with the appropriate toner and moisturizer, make a nice complete skin care gift. Bottle products in glass containers, such as French jelly jars, or small jars with cork tops. Label each cosmetic with a decorative sticker. Line a small basket with a brightly colored face cloth, sprinkle a few tablespoons of lavender, or rose petals along the bottom, and place your cosmetics inside. Tie a ribbon around the basket. Print complete instructions for each cosmetic on nice stationery and include it in an envelope or in scroll form with a ribbon. See Astringents and Toners (pages 23–30) for suggestion on how to bottle herbal tonics.

borax to dissolve in the herbal liquid. Both the wax/oil and the herbal liquid/borax mixtures should be approximately the same temperature when blending together. If one mixture is much warmer than the other, the end product may separate or feel lumpy or grainy.

Here's another hint: To make a product thicker or firmer, add more beeswax or cocoa butter. To soften, add more oil or herbal liquid and a pinch of borax.

ALOE AND CALENDULA CLEANSING LOTION

4 tablespoons (60 ml) avocado, sweet almond, castor,
  or grapeseed oil
1 tablespoon (15 ml) beeswax
1 tablespoon (15 ml) strong
  calendula or chamomile tea
2 tablespoons (30 ml) aloe
  vera gel
¼ teaspoon (1.25 ml) borax
50,000 international units
  vitamin A (capsules)
5 drops essential oil of carrot
  seed, sandalwood, marjoram, or geranium

Good for: normal and dry skin
Use: daily
Follow with: astringent or toner
Prep time: approximately 45 minutes
Mix with: whisk
Store in: low tub or jar
Yields: approximately 12 treatments
Special: Soothing and healing.

Melt together oil and beeswax in a small pan or double boil-er. Warm the tea and aloe vera gel in another pan and stir in borax until borax is dissolved. Remove both pans from heat and slowly pour the herbal mixture into the wax/oil pan, beating steadily with your whisk until cool, thick, and smooth. Pierce the vitamin A capsules and squeeze con-tents into lotion. Add essential oil. Blend completely one more time before storing. Use approximately 2 teaspoons (10 ml) per application. Does not require refrigeration if used up within 30 days, or unless weather is very hot.

BASIC COLD CREAM

1 ounce (30 ml) virgin olive, jojoba, sweet almond, apricot kernel, or avocado oil

4 ounces (120 ml) pure vegetable shortening (no lard, please!)

5 drops tincture of benzoin

5 drops of your favorite essential oil

Good for: normal and dry skin
Use: daily
Follow with: astringent/toner
Prep time: approximately 30 minutes
Mix with: whisk
Store in: low tub or jar
Yields: approximately 15 treatments
Special: Makes a great overnight treatment for hands or feet. Make sure you wear gloves or socks to bed!

Warm the oil and shortening in a small pan or double boiler until completely melted. Remove from heat and stir in the tincture of benzoin and essential oil. Allow to cool a bit, then begin whisking until cool, thick, and creamy. Store. Use approximately 2 teaspoons (10 ml) per application. Product performs best if used within 30 days; otherwise, refrigerate.

HERBAL SOAPY SKIN WASH

1 teaspoon (5 ml) sweet almond, jojoba, or grapeseed oil

5 drops essential oil of chamomile, German, or essential oil of sandalwood

3 drops essential oil of lemon balm (also called melissa)

5 drops essential oil of peppermint

5 drops essential oil of tea tree

16-ounce (500 ml) bottle plain castile liquid soap

Good for: normal and oily skin
Use: daily
Follow with: astringent or toner
Prep time: approximately 10 minutes
Mix with: shake before use
Store in: castile soap bottle
Yields: approximately 32 treatments
Special: This makes an especially invigorating body wash, too!

Add the drops of essential oils and teaspoon of oil to the bottle of castile soap. Shake vigorously. Use 1 tablespoon (15 ml) per application.

CLEANSING AND REJUVENATING OIL

2 tablespoons (30 ml)
each: melted coconut,
apricot kernel, avocado
or sunflower, grapeseed,
jojoba, sweet almond,
and virgin olive oils
5,000 international units
vitamin E oil
5 drops essential oil of
carrot seed, sandal-
wood, lavender, or
rosemary

Good for: all skin types
Use: daily
Follow with: astringent or toner
Prep time: 10 to 15 minutes
Mix with: spoon and small bowl
Store in: bottle
Yields: approximately 42 treatments
Special: Effectively removes eye makeup,
even stubborn waterproof types!

Combine all ingredients and store. Requires no refrigeration if used up within 30 days. Shake well before each use of approximately 1 teaspoon (5 ml) per application.

This special oil blend nourishes dry, parched skin and maintains the glow of normal, healthy skin. Oily skins can benefit from the nourishment of these healing oils, too, but make sure to apply the appropriate astringent following cleansing to remove any oil residue.

CLASSIC ROSEWATER AND GLYCERIN CLEANSER

½ cup (125 ml) rosewater
½ cup (125 ml) glycerin

Good for: normal and dry skin
Use: daily
Follow with: astringent and toner
Prep time: approximately 15 minutes
Mix with: shake before each use
Store in: bottle
Yields: 16 treatments
Special: Very gentle and soothing.

Combine ingredients and heat to just boiling. Do not allow to boil. Store. Apply this liquid cleanser with a washcloth or cotton pads. Use 1 tablespoon (15 ml) per application. Refrigeration not required.

LEMON CLEANSER

¼ cup (60 ml) plus 1 tablespoon (15 ml) grapeseed
  or apricot kernel oil
1 tablespoon (15 ml)
  beeswax
2 tablespoons (30 ml)
  strained lemon juice
¼ teaspoon (1.25 ml) borax
6 drops essential oil of
  lemon or tangerine

Good for: normal or oily skin
Use: daily
Follow with: astringent or toner
Prep time: approximately 45 minutes
Mix with: whisk
Store in: low tub or jar
Yields: approximately 9 treatments

In a small pan or double boiler, melt the oil and wax. Warm the lemon juice in another small pan and stir in borax until dissolved. Remove both pans from heat and slowly combine mixtures while beating steadily with your whisk until cool and creamy. Add essential oil and stir thoroughly. Store in refrigerator if not used up within 2 weeks or if house is very warm. Use 2 teaspoons (10 ml) per application.

STRAWBERRY CLEANSER

4 very ripe medium-sized
  strawberries, sliced
2 drops essential oil of
  yarrow or peppermint

Good for: normal or oily skin
Use: daily, when strawberries are in season
Follow with: astringent or toner
Prep time: 5 to 10 minutes
Mix with: mortar and pestle, spoon
Store in: Do not store. Mix only as needed.
Yields: 1 treatment
Special: The strawberry juice can also serve as a tooth cleanser and whitener. Very refreshing!

Mash the strawberries and press through mesh strainer or squeeze through cheesecloth or panty hose. Catch juice in a small condiment bowl. Add essential oil and stir to blend. Apply to face and neck with a saturated cotton square and massage with finger tips for about 1 minute. Avoid eye area. Rinse with cool water.

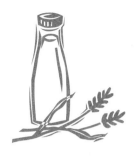

ASTRINGENTS AND TONERS

Astringents and toners, by definition, are agents used to remove the last traces of cleanser residue and also to remove excess perspiration and oil.

Astringents tend to be the stronger of the two and are usually used for normal-to-oily and oily skin types. Many commercial astringents contain alcohol and/or acetone (nail polish remover), which are very drying and damaging to the skin's surface. Herbal astringents tend to be gentler and are preferable to a chemical-based product.

Toners, on the other hand, perform the same function as an astringent but are designed for the normal-to-dry and dry skin. Thus, toners are milder by design and do not remove as much surface oil.

Storage tip: All of the following astringent and toner recipes should be stored in the refrigerator to preserve freshness unless otherwise indicated. Chemical preservatives have not been used in these recipes to extend the shelf life of the product. Please store your products in tightly sealed and labeled bottles or spritzers.

Application tip: Astringents and toners should be applied to the face and neck with a 100 percent cotton ball or pad in upward strokes. Always follow the use of these products with an appropriate moisturizer for your skin type.

GIFT IDEA

Who wouldn't appreciate receiving a freshly made herbal facial tonic packaged in a colored glass or decorative vinegar bottle topped with a cork? What a creative and useful gift! To make it even nicer, add a fresh sprig or peel of the herb called for in the recipe to the bottle. This just adds to the aesthetic appeal. Add a decorative label with instructions for use and make sure to note if it needs to be refrigerated.

LEMON REFRESHER

Juice of half a lemon
½ cup (125 ml) witch hazel
(commercially prepared
is fine)

Good for: oily skin
Use: daily
Follow with: moisturizer
Prep time: approximately 5 minutes
Mix with: cup or bowl and spoon
Store in: bottle or spritzer
Yields: approximately 24 treatments
Special: Very refreshing.

Mix ingredients, store, and shake well before each use. Use approximately 1 teaspoon (5 ml) per application.

PARSLEY AND PEPPERMINT ASTRINGENT

1 cup (250 ml) distilled
water
¼ cup (60 ml) fresh
chopped parsley
¼ cup (60 ml) fresh peppermint leaves or 2 table-
spoons (30 ml) dried
10 drops tincture of benzoin

Good for: normal and oily skin
Use: daily
Follow with: moisturizer
Prep time: approximately 35 minutes
Mix with: shake before use
Store in: bottle or spritzer
Yields: approximately 48 treatments

Bring water to boil and remove from heat. Add herbs and allow to steep for 30 minutes. Keep the lid on the pot while steeping. Add tincture of benzoin. Strain and store. Each week make a new solution. Use approximately 1 teaspoon (5 ml) per application.

pH RESTORER

~~~~~~~~

2 cups (500 ml) distilled
water
¼ cup (60 ml) apple cider
vinegar
10 drops favorite essential
oil — try lavender,
lemon, or rose

Good for: all skin types
Use: daily
Follow with: moisturizer
Prep time: approximately 5 to 10 minutes
Mix with: shake before use
Store in: bottle or spritzer
Yields: approximately 32 treatments
Special: Softens skin.

Combine ingredients and store. Use approximately 1 tablespoon (15 ml) per application. Splash it on if you wish. The vinegar will help combat the alkaline residue that soap or cleansers can leave behind. When your skin maintains the correct pH balance (5.5), it has a much better chance of fighting off infections. Requires no refrigeration.

OLD-FASHIONED LAVENDER TONER

~~~~~~~~

1 tablespoon (15 ml) lavender flowers
1 cup (250 ml) witch hazel
6 drops essential oil of
lavender

Good for: normal and dry skin
Use: daily
Follow with: moisturizer
Prep time: 2 weeks
Mix with: shake jar occasionally
during 2-week period
Store in: bottle or spritzer
Yields: approximately 48 treatments
Special: Smells sweet and floral.

Combine ingredients in a tightly lidded jar and store in a dark, cool place. Allow lavender to steep for 2 weeks. Shake jar vigorously every other day or so. Strain and bottle. Use approximately 1 teaspoon (5 ml) per application and shake well before each use. Requires no refrigeration.

FENNEL SOOTHER

2 cups (500 ml) distilled
  water
1 tablespoon (15 ml)
  crushed fennel seeds
2 teaspoons (10 ml)
  glycerin
¼ cup (60 ml) apple cider
  vinegar

Good for: all skin types, especially rashy and irritated
Use: daily
Follow with: moisturizer
Prep time: 50 to 55 minutes
Mix with: mortar and pestle to crush seeds
Store in: bottle or spritzer
Yields: approximately 32 treatments
Special: Softens skin and hair, if used as a rinse; restores pH.

Boil water. Remove from heat and add crushed fennel seeds. Let steep for 45 minutes. Strain, add glycerin and vinegar, and store. Shake well before each use. Use 1 tablespoon (15 ml) per application; splash on if desired. Does not require refrigeration if product is used up within 30 days.

ACNE ASTRINGENT

2 cups (500 ml) distilled
  water
1 tablespoon (15 ml) yarrow
1 tablespoon (15 ml) calendula or chamomile
15 drops tincture of
  benzoin
6 drops essential oil of
  peppermint

Good for: oily skin
Use: daily
Follow with: moisturizer
Prep time: approximately 35 minutes
Mix with: shake before use
Store in: bottle or spritzer
Yields: approximately 96 treatments
Special: Healing and soothing.

Boil water. Remove from heat and add herbs. Cover and steep for 30 minutes. Strain. Add tincture of benzoin and peppermint oil. Store. Use 1 teaspoon (5 ml) per application. Refrigerate.

ALOE VERA TONER

Pure aloe vera gel

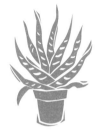

Good for: normal and oily skin (those with sensitive skin, see Note below)
Use: daily
Follow with: moisturizer
Prep time: none
Special: Great overall toner. Also relieves burns, sunburn, itch from insect bites.

Simply soak a cotton pad with the gel and use to freshen skin and remove excess oil. Follow directions on label regarding storage. If you use a leaf from your aloe plant, cut off the amount you are going to use and put the remainder of the leaf in a plastic bag and store in the refrigerator. Leaf will keep for about 3 days.

Note: Aloe juice may irritate sensitive skin. To lessen the irritating effects, dilute the gel 50/50 with distilled or spring water. Store in small jar and shake vigorously before application. Keep refrigerated.

TANGERINE TONER

½ cup (125 ml) witch hazel
6 drops essential oil of
    tangerine

Good for: normal and oily skin
Use: daily
Follow with: moisturizer
Prep time: 5 minutes
Mix with: shake before use
Store in: bottle or spritzer
Yields: approximately 24 treatments

Combine ingredients and shake vigorously. Store. Use 1 teaspoon (5 ml) per application. Requires no refrigeration.

HERBAL ASTRINGENT

1 cup (250 ml) distilled
  water
½ cup (125 ml) pure vodka
1 teaspoon (5 ml) each:
  sage, yarrow,
  chamomile, rosemary,
  lemon balm, peppermint,
  spearmint, and straw-
  berry leaves
¼ cup (60 ml) witch hazel

Good for: oily and normal skin
Use: daily
Follow with: moisturizer
Prep time: 2 weeks
Mix with: shake jar occasionally during
2-week period
Store in: bottle or spritzer
Yields: approximately 84 treatments
Special: Great following exercise!
Thoroughly removes all oil and perspiration.

Mix ingredients thoroughly and store for 2 weeks in a tightly sealed jar. Keep in a cool, dark place. Strain. Refrigeration is not required, though a cool product is nice on a hot summer day! Use 1 teaspoon (5 ml) per application.

MINTY ASTRINGENT

1 tablespoon (15 ml) fresh
  peppermint, spearmint,
  or lemon balm (if dried,
  use 1½ teaspoons
  (7.5 ml) of herb
1 cup (250 ml) witch hazel

Good for: normal and oily skin
Use: daily
Follow with: moisturizer
Prep time: 1 week
Mix with: shake jar occasionally during
the week
Store in: bottle or spritzer
Yields: approximately 48 treatments
Special: Has a nice fragrance. Could be
used by men as an aftershave.

Combine the ingredients in a jar with a tight-fitting lid. Allow herb to steep for 1 week. Strain. Use 1 teaspoon (5 ml) per application. Refrigeration not required.

ORANGE FLOWER TONER

1 cup (250 ml) distilled
water
1 tablespoon (15 ml) orange
flowers
1 teaspoon (5 ml) rose
petals
2 tablespoons (30 ml)
glycerin

Good for: normal and dry skin
Use: daily
Follow with: moisturizer if necessary
Prep time: 50 to 55 minutes
Mix with: spoon or whisk, small bowl
Store in: bottle or spritzer
Yields: approximately 54 treatments
Special: Very gentle and soothing.

Bring water to a boil and remove from heat. Add herbs and steep for 45 minutes in a covered pot. Strain. Slowly add glycerin, stirring constantly. Store. Use 1 teaspoon (5 ml) per application. Shake vigorously before each use.

ELDERFLOWER TONER

1 cup (250 ml) distilled
water
1 tablespoon (15 ml) elder-
flowers
1 tablespoon (15 ml)
glycerin
5 drops essential oil of
sandalwood or lavender
(optional)

Good for: normal and dry skin
Use: daily
Follow with: moisturizer if necessary
Prep time: 50 to 55 minutes
Mix with: spoon or whisk, small bowl
Store in: bottle or spritzer
Yields: approximately 50 treatments
Special: Super for extra dry skin, especially if oil of sandalwood is used.

Bring water to a boil and remove from heat. Add herb and steep for 45 minutes in a covered pot. Strain. Slowly add glycerin and essential oil, stirring constantly. Store. Use 1 teaspoon (5 ml) per application. Shake vigorously before each use.

SPICY AFTERSHAVE

2 cups (500 ml) witch
   hazel
1 sprig fresh rosemary
1 sprig fresh mint of choice
1 cinnamon stick
5 to 10 whole cloves
2 strips fresh orange peel
   cut into spirals
2 strips fresh lemon peel
   cut into spirals
15 drops tincture of
   benzoin

Good for: all skin types, except very dry
Use: daily or as desired
Follow with: moisturizer
Prep time: 2 weeks
Mix with: shake bottle gently every 2 days
Store in: decorative bottle
Yields: approximately 12 splashes
Special: When strained, can be used as a scented hair rinse for normal or oily dark hair.

Place all of the ingredients and tincture of benzoin in a decorative bottle with the witch hazel. Cap tightly and store for 2 weeks. Leave the herbs and other ingredients in the bottle. Smells delightful! Use approximately 2½ tablespoons (37.5 ml) per application, or more if you like.

Note: Use organically grown fruit — if available — to avoid pesticide residue. Be sure to wash fruit thoroughly.

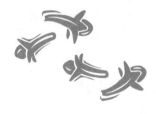

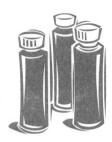

MOISTURIZING CREAMS AND LOTIONS

Moisturizers can be your skin's best friend! By applying a moisturizer to your skin, you are, in effect, putting a barrier between your skin and a world full of pollutants, drying air-conditioning and heat in your home or office, and the aging effects of the sun. Always use a moisturizer designed for your skin type, otherwise your skin may look oily from over-moisturizing or be thirsty from under-moisturizing.

Application tip: Moisturizers should always be applied following the use of your toner or astringent and immediately following a facial treatment, such as a scrub, steam, or mask. Apply your moisturizer onto a freshly cleansed face that is still slightly damp from the toner, astringent, or rinse water. Using upward, circular motions, apply your moisturizer the same way as you would your cleanser. Wait one minute to allow your skin to "drink" the moisture, then proceed with your makeup or sunscreen. The moisturizer "seals in" the moisture already present on your skin and thus prevents your delicate facial tissue from dehydrating. By all means, don't forget to moisturize your neck and chest. Many women neglect these areas, which can actually reveal the aging effects of sun exposure and general neglect sooner than your face. Moisturizing is the last step in your skin care process.

Important "cooking" instructions: Please read this section detailed under Cleansing Creams and Lotions (pages 18–19) before you proceed with the following recipes.

GIFT IDEA

Creams and lotions are a welcome treat any time of the year — especially during the summer and winter.

Make up a fresh batch of cream or lotion for a friend. Put it in an attractive glass or plastic jar and attach a label with instructions. Wrap it in tissue paper and place in a small gift bag. Include a pair of inexpensive cotton gloves or socks, especially if you make one of the heavier moisturizers that doubles as an overnight hand and foot conditioner.

"There is a case for keeping wrinkles. They are the long-service stripes earned in the hard campaign of life."

—editorial, *The London Daily Mail*

COCOA BUTTER LOTION FOR FACE AND BODY

1 tablespoon (15 ml) cocoa
butter
1 tablespoon (15 ml) anhydrous lanolin
⅔ cup (160 ml) grapeseed,
sweet almond, apricot
kernel, or jojoba oil
3 tablespoons (45 ml)
distilled water
½ teaspoon (2.5 ml) borax
6 drops essential oil of
sandalwood, fennel, or
geranium

Good for: normal and dry skin
Use: daily
Prep time: approximately 45 minutes
Mix with: whisk
Store in: low tub or jar
Yields: approximately 25 treatments,
depending on use

Melt together the cocoa butter, anhydrous lanolin, and oil in a small pan or double boiler. Heat the water in a separate pan and stir in borax until dissolved. Remove both from heat and slowly combine the mixtures, stirring with your whisk. Blend until cool and creamy. Add essential oil and blend again. Store. Use 2 or more teaspoons (10 ml) per application. Refrigeration not required if used up within 30 days.

LIGHT MOISTURIZER

½ cup (125 ml) distilled
water
3 teaspoons (15 ml)
glycerin
5 drops essential oil of
lemon

Good for: normal and oily skin
Use: daily
Prep time: approximately 5 minutes
Mix with: shake before use
Store in: bottle or spritzer
Yields: approximately 24 treatments

Pour ingredients into storage bottle and shake vigorously. Product can be applied using a cotton ball or by spraying the skin lightly and allowing to dry. Great to use anytime your skin needs refreshing or is feeling dehydrated. Use 1 teaspoon (5 ml) per application. Refrigeration not required.

PROTECTION CREAM

¼ cup (60 ml) pre-warmed coconut oil

½ cup (125 ml) sweet almond, extra-virgin olive, jojoba, or grape-seed oil

½ tablespoon (7.5 ml) cocoa butter

Good for: normal, dry, and severely chapped skin

Use: as desired

Prep time: approximately 45 minutes

Mix with: whisk

Store in: low tub or jar

Yields: approximately 12 treatments

Special: Can be used as an intensive overnight hand and foot cream.

Combine all ingredients in a small pan or double boiler and heat just until the cocoa butter melts. Remove from heat. Allow mixture to cool slightly, then beat vigorously, cool a bit more, then beat again until creamy.

I use this cream mainly on my body, especially on areas that need extra attention. In the winter, I take a warm bath, pat dry, slather this cream on generously everywhere, then put on my long flannel gown and socks and go to bed. My husband doesn't find this outfit attractive, by any means, but he does like the way my skin feels the next morning. Use 1 tablespoon (15 ml), more or less, per application. No need to refrigerate if used up within 30 days.

Note: Cream may harden in cold weather. To soften, place container in a shallow pan of hot water for about 10 minutes.

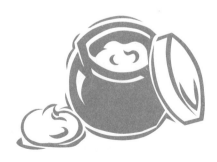

BABY'S BOTTOM CREAM

2 teaspoons (10 ml) non-petroleum jelly

2 teaspoons (10 ml) cocoa butter

2 tablespoons (30 ml) grapeseed, jojoba, or castor oil

2 drops essential oil of orange blossom, apple blossom, carrot seed, or lemon balm (melissa)

Good for: all skin types, especially normal and dry

Use: as desired

Prep time: approximately 30 minutes

Mix with: whisk

Store in: low tub or jar

Yields: approximately 8 treatments

Special: Makes a great "ski cream"! Really protects against dry, frigid air. Also makes a good diaper rash prevention cream.

Heat all ingredients (except essential oil) in a small pan just until the cocoa butter is melted. Remove from heat and allow to cool a bit, then stir occasionally until cool and thick. Add essential oil, then beat again. Store. This cream will not turn white but will be relatively thick and clear. Use 1 teaspoon (5 ml) per application. Refrigeration not required.

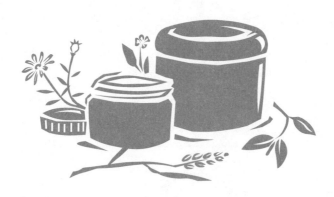

MASKS

The use of masks dates back to ancient civilizations that believed particular types of mud and clay, when applied to the body, had healing properties. Many tribes used clay that was tinted various colors. These specially prepared clays were painted onto the faces and bodies of tribe members to signify a particular event, such as a celebration or a war, was about to take place. Today masks are used to deep-clean, tone, or soften the skin, depending on the ingredients they contain.

Masks can be made from natural ingredients, such as fuller's earth, French clay, or brewer's yeast, which absorb excess oil and dead cells from the skin's surface and stimulate a sluggish complexion. Masks can also be made from fresh, ripe peaches and cream, which moisturize a dry complexion and leave your skin with a wonderful "peaches and cream" glow. Set aside some personal time each week to devote to your skin. Relax and enjoy one of the following recipes. Your mind will appreciate the quiet time, and your skin will reward you with a renewed complexion!

Application tip: Masks should always be applied to freshly cleansed, damp skin. Begin at the neck and apply in an upward action. Avoid applying the mask to the delicate eye area, as irritation may develop. Allow the mask to remain on your skin at least 20 minutes or longer, unless otherwise specified. Remove with a warm, wet washcloth, and apply moisturizer if necessary.

GIFT IDEA

There are several mask recipes that can be packaged and given as gifts. These include masks which are based on dry ingredients, such as clay, ground oatmeal, sunflower seed meal, wheat germ, brewer's yeast, and almond meal. Prepare a few of the base ingredients and measure approximately ½ cup (125 ml) of each and put into individual plastic bags, tightly sealed. Attach instructions for the mask to each bag with a ribbon. Place three or four bags inside a decorative tin or small wooden box.

BASIC CLAY MASK

½ cup (125 ml) French clay
   or fuller's earth
Cream — dry skin
Milk — normal skin
Water — oily skin

Good for: all skin types

Use: one to two times per week, or as desired

Follow with: moisturizer

Prep time: approximately 5 minutes

Mix with: small bowl and spoon

Store in: dry ingredient only — low tub/jar, zip-seal bag, or tin

Yields: approximately 8 treatments

Combine 1 tablespoon (15 ml) of clay with enough of the appropriate liquid (determined by your skin type) to form a smooth, spreadable paste. Spread onto face and neck and allow to dry thoroughly. Rinse.

This mask can serve as an overnight pimple treatment. Take a cotton swab and apply a dab on each pimple and leave on overnight. In the morning, rinse the remaining bits of mask with warm water. The clay absorbs the excess oil overnight and aids in the healing of the pimples.

EGG WHITE FIRMING MASK

White of 1 fresh egg
1 teaspoon (5 ml)
   cornstarch

Good for: normal and oily skin, especially skin with large pores

Use: one time per week, or as desired

Follow with: moisturizer

Prep time: 5 to 10 minutes

Mix with: small bowl and whisk

Store in: Do not store. Mix as needed.

Yields: 1 treatment

Special: Minimizes the appearance of large pores. Excellent skin tightener.

Combine the ingredients and beat until stiff peaks form. Smooth onto a clean face and allow to dry. Rinse. If you have a slant board, lie on this while your mask is drying. You'll swear you've had a mini face-lift when you're finished!

YOGURT ASTRINGENT/BLEACHING MASK

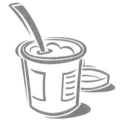

2 teaspoons (10 ml) plain
   yogurt

Good for: normal, oily, and blotchy skin
Use: one to two times per week, or as
desired
Follow with: moisturizer
Prep time: approximately 1 minute
Mix with: small bowl and spoon
Store in: keep yogurt refrigerated
Yields: 1 treatment
Special: Great for a fading tan, slightly
bleaches and evens skin tone with
repeated use.

Apply the yogurt to face and neck. Allow to dry, preferably while lying
down. Rinse.

BREWER'S YEAST MASK

1 tablespoon (15 ml) brewer's yeast
1 tablespoon (15 ml) milk or
   water

Good for: normal and oily skin
Use: one to two times per week
Follow with: moisturizer
Prep time: approximately 5 minutes
Mix with: small bowl and spoon
Store in: Do not store. Mix only as needed.
Yields: 1 treatment
Special: Brings a rosy glow to the skin.
Helps chase away that winter "pasty
pale" look.

Combine ingredients to form a smooth paste. You may need more or less
liquid than called for, depending on the brand of yeast used. Spread onto
face in a thin layer, allow to dry, rinse. This mask may tingle as it dries.
This is normal. If it starts to sting, rinse it off immediately and apply a
good moisturizer.

PAPAYA "NO-MORE-PORES"
DOUBLE MASK TREATMENT

¼ cup (60 ml) freshly
   mashed papaya
1 teaspoon (5 ml) fresh
   pineapple juice
   (optional)

Good for: all skin types, except sensitive
and sunburned
Use: one time per week
Follow with: moisturizer
Prep time: 5 to 10 minutes
Mix with: mortar and pestle, or small
bowl and fork
Store in: Do not store. Mix as needed.
Yields: 1 treatment
Special: Mask is slightly bleaching and
leaves a wonderful glow upon the skin.

Mask #1

Mash the papaya and combine with the pineapple juice (if available) until
thoroughly mixed and smooth. Gently pat this onto face and neck. Try to
lie down and rest while this mask is doing its job. You may want to place
a towel around your head and behind your neck as this mask can be a bit
runny. Your face will probably tingle a bit — relax, it just means the ingredients are working properly. Rinse.

The papaya and pineapple contain an enzyme which helps to dissolve
and lift away dry skin scales which can, over time, build up on your skin
and leave a dull appearance.

Mask #2

Now apply the basic clay mask (see recipe, page 36) using strong sage or
rosemary tea in place of the milk, cream, or water to mix with the clay. *If
your skin is especially sensitive, use cream as your liquid.* Apply as directed. Dry skin types may want to apply a thin layer of moisturizer first,
then proceed with the clay mask. All skin types should apply moisturizer after the second mask.

Results: After you've applied your moisturizer, look closely at your
face. It should look smoother and more refined. I do this treatment as
often as I can when I can get fresh, ripe papaya and pineapple.

HONEY AND WHEAT GERM SOFTENING MASK

1 tablespoon (15 ml) fresh
 honey
1 teaspoon (5 ml) wheat
 germ
1 teaspoon (5 ml) sunflower
 seed meal

Good for: normal and dry skin
Use: as desired
Follow with: moisturizer, if necessary
Prep time: approximately 5 minutes
Mix with: small bowl and spoon
Store in: Do not store. Mix as needed.
Yields: 1 treatment
Special: Leaves skin soft and moist.

Thoroughly combine all ingredients in a small bowl and allow to set for 1 minute. Pat onto face and neck. Leave on for approximately 30 minutes and rinse after with a very warm damp cloth.

DEEP PORE CLEANSER

1 teaspoon (5 ml) almond
 meal
1 teaspoon (5 ml) sunflower
 seed meal
1 teaspoon (5 ml) ground
 oatmeal
¼ teaspoon (1.25 ml)
 quality vegetable oil
¼ medium-sized ripe toma-
 to or 1-inch chunk of
 cucumber, peeled
water

Good for: normal and oily skin
Use: one to two times per week
Follow with: moisturizer
Prep time: 10 to 15 minutes
Mix with: blender, small bowl and spoon
Store in: Do not store. Mix as needed.
Yields: 1 treatment
Special: This recipe can double as a facial scrub.

Place tomato or cucumber into a blender and add a small amount of water, one tablespoon at most. Blend until smooth. Strain. Combine enough of the vegetable liquid with the meal and oil to form a smooth paste. Spread onto face and neck, allow to dry, rinse.

"PEACHES AND CREAM" GLOW MASK

½ very ripe small peach
   (peeled)
1 tablespoon (15 ml) heavy
   cream

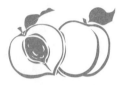

Good for: normal-to-very dry, and sensitive skin

Use: as desired

Follow with: moisturizer, if necessary

Prep time: approximately 5 minutes

Mix with: mortar and pestle, or small bowl and fork

Store in: Do not store. Mix as needed.

Yields: 1 treatment

Special: Highly moisturizing and fragrant.

Mash the peach half and combine with cream until smooth. Apply mixture to face and neck and leave on for 30 minutes while lying down or reclining on a slant board. Rinse. This mask is as delicious as it is nourishing for your skin. You may be tempted to mix up a larger quantity (made with milk instead of cream), add a dab of honey, and drink it for lunch!

Note: Mask can be runny. You may wish to wrap a towel around your hair to catch any drips.

APPLESAUCE AND WHEAT GERM MOISTURIZING MASK

1 tablespoon (15 ml) fresh
   applesauce
1 tablespoon (15 ml) raw
   wheat germ
2 teaspoons (10 ml) oil of
   wheat germ, jojoba, or
   sweet almond

Good for: normal and dry skin

Use: as desired

Follow with: moisturizer, if necessary

Prep time: approximately 10 minutes

Mix with: small bowl and spoon

Store in: Do not store. Mix as needed.

Yields: 1 treatment

Special: Leaves skin moist and rosy.

Mix the applesauce and wheat germ thoroughly. Allow mixture to thicken for 5 minutes or until the wheat germ absorbs some of the apple juice. Apply to face and throat. This is another mask that can be a bit messy, so you may wish to wrap your hair with a towel. Rinse. Follow with an oil facial massage. Massage the oil onto your face and throat in gentle, circular motions for 5 minutes. Towel dry. Your face should be warm and glowing!

HONEY MASSAGE MASK

2 to 3 teaspoons (10 to
15 ml) fresh honey
Hair pins or shower cap

Good for: all skin types, especially dehydrated and/or flaky
Use: as desired
Follow with: moisturizer, if necessary
Prep time: two to three minutes
Yields: 1 treatment
Special: Softens and moisturizes.

Apply a thin coat of your favorite honey to your entire face and neck. Be sure to pull your hair up and off your face. When honey is spread evenly, it will bead up as water beads up on your car after a shower. Leave on for 15 minutes while you lie down and rest. Your skin will begin to feel very warm and relaxed. Don't fall asleep!

Before rinsing, begin to gently pat your entire face with your fingertips. Make quick tapping motions like you are playing the piano. Do this for about 5 minutes. Rinse with very warm water and a damp cloth.

AVOCADO AND BUTTERMILK MASK

¼ very ripe avocado
Buttermilk

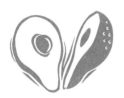

Good for: normal-to-very dry, especially rough or chapped skin
Use: as desired
Follow with: moisturizer, if necessary
Prep time: approximately 5 minutes
Mix with: small bowl and fork
Store in: Do not store. Mix as needed.
Yields: 1 treatment
Special: A larger batch can be made and applied to dry hair to serve as a conditioner for normal and dry hair. Leave on for 30 minutes. Rinse and shampoo out.

Mash together the avocado and just enough buttermilk to form a creamy paste. Apply in upward strokes to face and throat. If possible, lie in the sun to allow the oils of the avocado to warm and penetrate your skin. Rinse after 20 to 30 minutes. Your skin should feel velvety soft.

OATMEAL MASK

4 teaspoons (20 ml)
ground oatmeal
4 teaspoons (20 ml) milk
or buttermilk

Good for: all skin types
Use: as desired
Follow with: moisturizer, if necessary
Prep time: approximately 5 minutes
Mix with: small bowl and spoon
Store in: Do not store. Mix as needed.
Yields: 1 treatment
Special: Mask has a slight bleaching effect if used repeatedly. Helps even out a fading tan.

Combine ingredients and allow to thicken for a few minutes. Spread onto face, throat, and chest area. Relax on a slant board if possible, or just recline until dry. Rinse.

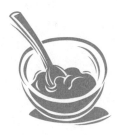

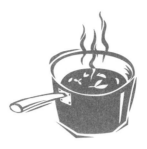

FACIAL STEAMS

An herbal facial steam will soften the skin and allow the pores to perspire and breathe. As the steam penetrates the skin, the various herbs will soften the skin's surface, act as an astringent and/or aid in healing skin lesions. Also, any clogging from dirt or makeup will be loosened for easy removal afterward.

Herbal steams may be used regularly by those with normal, dry, or oily skins. Those of you with sensitive skin or thread veins, however, should abstain.

Always cleanse your skin before steaming.

Preparation: To prepare for a facial steam, boil 3 cups (750 ml) of distilled water. If a recipe calls for vinegar, boil it with the water. Remove from heat and add the herbs to steep, with the lid on the pot, for about 5 minutes. Now, place the pot of herbs in a safe, stable place where you can sit comfortably for 10 minutes. Use a bath towel to create a tent over your head, shoulders, and steaming herb pot. With your eyes closed, breathe deeply and relax as you cleanse your pores with this wonderful, fragrant steam.

Important note: Please allow 8 to 10 inches between the steaming herb pot and your face so you won't risk burning your skin.

After your skin has been "steam cleaned," rinse with tepid water first, then follow with cool splashes. Pat skin until almost dry. Following a facial steam is the ideal time to use a mask and moisturizer so that your skin may benefit from a full treatment. Enjoy!

GIFT IDEA

An attractive container to use when giving a freshly made facial steam recipe is a one-quart size, blue or red speckled enameled pot. You can find these in many discount stores or specialty kitchen shops. Make up about ½ cup (125 ml) of the herb mixture from one of the following recipes, put it in a plastic freezer bag, tie with a ribbon, and attach instructions and a measuring spoon. Place this inside the pot (which is to be used to make the facial steam). A nice accompaniment is a bath towel. If you can, choose a towel and pot that are the same color.

Special note: If you would like to make up a larger batch of your favorite facial steam mixture to have handy, store the dry ingredients in an airtight zip-seal bag, low tub or jar, or tin, and keep in a dark, cool place. If the recipe calls for added oil or vinegar, add these when you are ready to do a facial steam.

What can you do with the leftover herbal liquid after you have steamed your face? Let it cool and use it to water your plants, strain it and add it to your bath water, or pour the whole mixture onto your compost pile. Don't waste it! Do not, however, pour a vinegar solution on your plants.

BASIC STEAM

3 cups (750 ml) distilled water
1 teaspoon (5 ml) calendula (marigold)
1 teaspoon (5 ml) chamomile
1 teaspoon (5 ml) raspberry leaves
1 teaspoon (5 ml) peppermint
1 teaspoon (5 ml) strawberry leaves

Good for: all skin types
Use: one to two times per week
Follow with: moisturizer
Prep time: approximately 15 minutes
Store in: Dry ingredients: zip-seal bag, low tub or jar, tin. Keep in cool, dark place.
Yields: 1 treatment
Special: Can double as a hair rinse for light brown and blonde/red hair. Strain before using.

Follow this steam up with a mask if you wish, followed by moisturizer.

REFRESHING PORE CLEANSER

3 cups (750 ml) distilled
   water
1 teaspoon (5 ml) yarrow
1 teaspoon (5 ml) sage or
   rosemary
1 teaspoon (5 ml) pepper-
   mint

Good for: normal and oily skin
Use: one to two times per week
Follow with: moisturizer
Prep time: approximately 15 minutes
Store in: Dry ingredients: zip-seal bag, low tub or jar, tin. Keep in cool, dark place.
Yields: 1 treatment

Rinse with tepid water, then cool. Follow this steam with a mask, followed by moisturizer.

pH RESTORER

3 cups (750 ml) distilled
   water
½ cup (125 ml) apple cider
   vinegar
1 teaspoon (5 ml) lavender
   flowers or rosemary
1 teaspoon (5 ml) rose
   petals

Good for: all skin types
Use: one to two times per week
Follow with: moisturizer
Prep time: approximately 15 minutes
Store in: Dry ingredients: zip-seal bag, low tub or jar, tin. Keep in cool, dark place.
Yields: 1 treatment
Special: Softens skin.

This facial steam is particularly good if you wear makeup daily or use soap to cleanse your skin. Most makeup and soap leave an alkaline residue on your skin which leaves it wide open for bacterial infection, pimples, and patchy dryness. Your skin is naturally a bit on the acid side with a pH of approximately 5.5. The vinegar in this steam helps restore your skin's proper pH balance.

After completing this steam, use a mask, followed by moisturizer.

DRY SKIN SAUNA

3 cups (750 ml) distilled
  water
1 teaspoon (5 ml) orange
  peel or orange flowers
1 teaspoon (5 ml) comfrey
  leaves
1 teaspoon (5 ml) elder
  flowers
1 teaspoon (5 ml) sweet
  almond or avocado oil
  (any quality vegetable
  oil will do)

Good for: normal and dry skin
Use: one to two times per week
Follow with: moisturizer
Prep time: approximately 15 minutes
Store in: Dry ingredients: zip-seal bag,
low tub or jar, tin. Keep in cool dark place.
Yields: 1 treatment
Special: Can double as a toner. Strain and
cool. Store and refrigerate. Shake before
each use.

This steam treatment works especially well when followed by a mask and moisturizer.

WRINKLE CHASER

3 cups (750 ml) distilled
  water
1 tablespoon (15 ml)
  crushed fennel seed
2 drops essential oil of
  rose

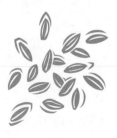

Good for: all skin types, especially
dehydrated, rough, and chapped
Use: one to two times per week
Follow with: moisturizer
Prep time: 10 to 15 minutes
Mix with: mortar and pestle to crush seeds
Store in: Dry ingredients: zip-seal bag,
low tub or jar, tin. Keep in cool dark place.
Yields: 1 treatment
Special: Soothes and softens skin. This
mixture, when strained and cooled, can be
used as a soothing facial splash, mouth-
wash, or softening hair rinse. Refrigerate
any unused portion.

Follow this treatment up with a mask and moisturizer.

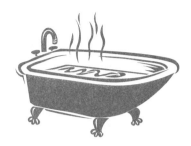

BODY BATHS

Bathing has been an important daily ritual for thousands of years. The bath is not for hygienic purposes alone, but can also be used for pampering the body and spirit. Cleopatra was known for her soothing milk baths and Marie Antoinette for her long, luxurious herbal ones. Healing treatments can be incorporated into the bathing ritual, too. Health spas the world over offer mineral baths in hot springs, sulfur waters, and mud (used to remove impurities from the skin). Various herbal and salt baths are also enjoyable for their fragrant and soothing benefits.

Whether you're interested in soaking your tired, aching muscles and daily tensions away, stimulating your circulation, soothing your dry skin, or enjoying a calming bath laced with essential oil of gardenia, these recipes are sure to please.

Shower fanatics beware: Try a few of these tub-tantalizing mixtures and you may become a true bath lover after all!

Special tip: Keep your bath water warm, not hot. Hot water causes your skin to perspire and will not enable your body to absorb the properties of the natural ingredients you choose to include in your bath. Also, the hotter the water, the quicker the essential oils dissipate into the air and lose their qualities, and hot water dehydrates your skin.

GIFT IDEA

Bath salts are an easy-to-make, inexpensive, and warmly welcomed gift. Make up a large batch of the Herbal Bath Salts recipe (see page 49), enough for about four baths, in a large bowl. Find a decorative tin or jar with a tight-fitting lid and fill with the bath salts. (You might want to put a small muslin bag of rice in the bottom to absorb any moisture that might find its way into the container.) Wrap the container in plain brown paper and gather at the top with ribbon or twine and attach a hand-printed card detailing the instructions.

HERBAL BATH BAG

2 tablespoons (30 ml) elder
    flowers, chamomile, laven-
    der, lemon balm, or jasmine
1 tablespoon (15 ml)
    raspberry leaves
1 tablespoon (15 ml)
    comfrey leaves
1 tablespoon (15 ml) ground
    oatmeal
8-inch x 8-inch square of
    muslin, cheese cloth,
    or foot of an old nylon
    stocking
String or yarn

Good for: all skin types
Use: as desired
Follow with: moisturize body after bath
Prep time: 10 to 15 minutes
Store in: Several bags could be made and stored in a zip-seal bag, low tub or jar, or tin.
Yields: 1 treatment
Special: Softens and soothes skin, pleasant scent.

Place herbs and oatmeal in center of cloth or toe of stocking. Gather into a pouch and tie with a string long enough to hang from the hot water tap in the tub to allow the running water to flow through. After the tub is full, untie the bag from the tap and let it float around in the water. Sit back and enjoy! Discard when finished.

SKIN SOFTENING WASH BAG

¼ cup (60 ml) ground
    oatmeal
¼ cup (60 ml) ground
    sunflower seeds
8-inch x 8-inch square of
    muslin, cheese cloth, or
    foot of an old nylon
    stocking
String or yarn

Good for: normal and dry skin
Use: as desired
Follow with: moisturize body after bath
Prep time: 5 to 10 minutes
Store in: Several bags could be made and stored in a zip-seal bag, jar, or tin.
Yields: 1 treatment
Special: Softens and moisturizes skin.

Place ingredients in center of cloth or toe of stocking. Gather into a pouch and tie with a short string. As you relax in the tub, gently rub your entire body with the bag, then let it remain in the water releasing its softening properties. Discard bag when finished.

MILK BATH

½ cup (125 ml) powdered whole milk
1 tablespoon (15 ml) apricot kernel, castor, jojoba, grapeseed, or quality vegetable oil
8 drops essential oil of chamomile, jasmine, lavender, rosemary, or marjoram

Good for: normal and dry skin
Use: as desired
Follow with: moisturize body after bath, if necessary
Prep time: approximately 5 minutes
Store in: Do not store. Make as needed.
Yields: 1 treatment
Special: Leaves skin feeling silky soft.

Pour powdered milk and tablespoon of oil together directly under running bath water. Add essential oil immediately before stepping into tub. Swish with hands to mix. Now relax!

HERBAL BATH SALTS

½ cup (125 ml) baking soda
½ cup (125 ml) sea salt
15 drops essential oil of clary sage, marjoram, lavender, or sandalwood

Good for: all skin types, especially itchy and rashy skin
Use: as desired
Follow with: moisturize body after bath
Prep time: approximately 5 minutes
Store in: A larger amount of bath salts can be made and stored in a zip-seal bag, low tub, jar, or tin.
Yields: 1 treatment
Special: Softens and smoothes rough skin.

Turn on the tap full blast and pour soda and salt mixture into tub. Add essential oil when tub is full and swish water to mix.

SORE MUSCLE SOAK

½ cup (125 ml) Epsom
   salts
½ cup (125 ml) baking soda
1 tablespoon (15 ml) sage
1 tablespoon (15 ml)
   marjoram
1 tablespoon (15 ml)
   chamomile
1 tablespoon (15 ml) pine
   needles
2 teaspoons (10 ml) lemon
   balm
2 teaspoons (10 ml)
   peppermint
10 drops essential oil of
   eucalyptus, peppermint,
   or juniper
10-inch x 10-inch square of
   muslin, cheesecloth, or
   foot of an old nylon
   stocking
String or yarn

Good for: all skin types
Use: following exercise, or as desired
Follow with: moisturize body after bath
Prep time: approximately 15 minutes
Store in: Several bags could be made and stored in a zip-seal bag, jar, or tin.
Yields: 1 treatment
Special: Helps relax tense, sore muscles. The fragrance will soothe frayed nerves.

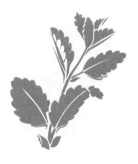

Place all ingredients in center of cloth and tie into a bag. When adding essential oil, allow the drops to be absorbed by the baking soda before tying the bag. Tie beneath the tap and allow the running water to flow through. When tub is full, remove bag from tap and massage your body with it for a few minutes, then let it float in the tub. Discard after use.

VINEGAR BATH

3 cups (750 ml) apple
  cider vinegar
½ cup (125 ml) rosemary or
  juniper berries; either
  herb may be cut 50/50
  with comfrey

Good for: all skin types, except very sensitive
Use: as desired
Follow with: moisturize body after bath
Prep time: 3 to 4 hours
Store in: decorative glass jar or any glass container
Yields: approximately 3 treatments
Special: Soothes and softens itchy skin. Good to use in a foot bath, too.

In a pan, heat vinegar to boiling. Remove from heat and add herbs. Cover and allow to steep for several hours. Strain and store in a pretty container. Use 1 cup per bath. Add liquid to bath while tap is running.

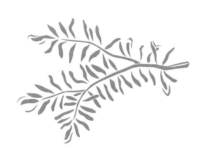

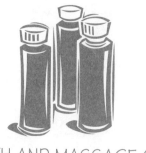

BATH AND MASSAGE OILS

Bath and massage oils are very easy to make at home. You simply need a base oil and any essential oil you desire. I like to use jojoba oil as my base because it does not need refrigeration and will not go rancid. Grapeseed oil makes a great base for massage oil because it is very light and leaves the skin soft, not greasy.

GIFT IDEA

Bath and massage oils are a great treatment for dry skin. In addition, scented oils can be mentally relaxing, stimulating, or can be used to create a sensual mood.

Bath oils make the perfect gift for a friend or loved one who has a particularly stressful lifestyle and enjoys unwinding with a long, luxurious bath. Massage oils (and the accompanying massage) are a great treat for special friends and spouses.

Package oils in blue, green, or brown glass bottles to protect the essential oil from the light. Decorative bottles can be found in antique stores, at flea markets, as well as at bath and gift shops. Make sure the lids fit tightly! Attach a gift card with your personalized message.

NOURISHING OIL

1 tablespoon (15 ml) each
of the following oils:
sweet almond, virgin
olive, avocado, jojoba,
apricot kernel, and
grapeseed
1,200 international units
vitamin E oil (d-alpha
tocopherol)

Good for: all skin types, especially normal and dry
Use: as desired
Follow with: moisturize body after bath, if necessary
Oily skin: apply astringent to body, if desired
Prep time: approximately 10 minutes
Mix with: shake before use
Store in: bottle
Yields: approximately 10 treatments, for bath
Special: A good mixture to rub into cuticles, especially if dry and ragged.

Combine ingredients in a bottle. Tightly cap and shake vigorously. Store in refrigerator. For bath, add 2 teaspoons (10 ml) to running water. For massage, use as needed.

FLORAL OIL

¾ cup (180 ml) jojoba oil
½ teaspoon (2.5 ml)
essential oil of rose
½ teaspoon (2.5 ml)
essential oil of lavender
1 teaspoon (5 ml) essen-
tial oil of geranium
¼ teaspoon (1.25 ml)
essential oil of ylang-
ylang

Good for: normal and dry skin
Use: as desired
Follow with: moisturize body, if necessary
Prep time: 5 to 10 minutes
Mix with: shake before use
Store in: bottle
Yields: approximately 18 treatments, for bath
Special: Softens skin and leaves a romantic floral fragrance upon it.

Mix together the jojoba oil and essential oil, store in a tightly sealed bottle, in a dark place. Add 2 teaspoons (10 ml) oil to bath while tub is filling. For massage, use ½ teaspoon (2.5 ml) essential oil to ½ cup (125 ml) jojoba oil.

To make a glorious floral perfume: Mix the essential oils only, in a beautiful, tiny bottle. Cap tightly and shake well. Apply just a touch on your pulse points: neck, wrists, and behind knees.

STIMULATING HERBAL OIL

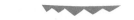

¾ cup (180 ml) jojoba oil
2 teaspoons (10 ml) of
   any combination of the
   following essential oils:
   basil, bay, eucalyptus,
   lavender, lemon, lemongrass, any of the
   mints, rosemary,
   tangerine, pine

Good for: all skin types, especially normal and dry
Use: as desired
Follow with: moisturize body after bath, if necessary
Oily skin: apply astringent to body, if desired
Prep time: approximately 10 minutes
Mix with: shake before use
Store in: bottle
Yields: approximately 18 treatments, for bath
Special: A good mixture to rub into cuticles, especially if dry and ragged.

Combine oils, store in a tightly sealed bottle in a dark place. Add 2 teaspoons (10 ml) to running bath water. For massage, use ½ teaspoon (2.5 ml) essential oil to ½ cup (125 ml) jojoba oil.

UPLIFTING OIL

3 teaspoons (15 ml)
   jojoba oil
2 drops each, essential
   oils of chamomile, peppermint, rosemary,
   juniper, and eucalyptus

Good for: normal and dry skin
Use: as desired
Follow with: moisturize body, if necessary
Prep time: approximately 5 minutes
Yields: 1 treatment
Special: Makes an excellent refreshing and energizing bath oil or deodorizing massage oil for the feet.

Add to bath while tap is running. For foot massage, combine ingredients in a small bowl and have a friend massage your clean, tired feet for 15 minutes, put on socks, and go to bed.

EXOTIC OIL

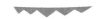

¾ cup (180 ml) jojoba oil
½ teaspoon (2.5 ml)
   essential oil of sandalwood
½ teaspoon (2.5 ml)
   essential oil of patchouli
½ teaspoon (2.5 ml) musk
   oil, synthetic
¼ teaspoon (1.25 ml)
   essential oil of vetivert

Good for: normal and dry skin
Use: as desired
Follow with: moisturize body, if necessary
Prep time: 5 to 10 minutes
Mix with: shake before use
Store in: bottle
Yields: approximately 18 treatments, for bath
Special: Softens skin and leaves a sensual, musky fragrance upon it.

Mix together the jojoba oil and essential oil, store in a tightly sealed bottle, in a dark place. Add 2 teaspoons (10 ml) oil to bath while tub is filling. For massage, use ½ teaspoon (2.5 ml) essential oil to ½ cup (125 ml) jojoba oil.

For an exotic perfume: Mix the essential oils only and bottle.

RELAXING OIL

¾ cup (180 ml) jojoba oil
2 teaspoons (10 ml) of any
   of the following essential oils: chamomile,
   clary sage, marjoram,
   sandalwood, geranium,
   ylang-ylang, or jasmine

Good for: normal and dry skin
Use: as desired
Follow with: moisturize body, if necessary
Prep time: approximately 5 minutes
Mix with: shake before use
Store in: bottle
Yields: approximately 18 treatments, for bath
Special: Softens skin. Fragrance helps relieve stress.

Mix together the jojoba oil and essential oil, store in a tightly sealed bottle, in a dark place. Add 2 teaspoons (10 ml) oil to bath while tub is filling. For massage, use ½ teaspoon (2.5 ml) essential oil to ½ cup (125 ml) jojoba oil.

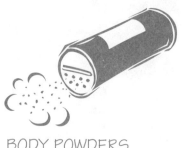

BODY POWDERS

When you think of body powder, the first ingredient that comes to mind is talc, right? Talc is inexpensive but can irritate your lungs and frequently contains traces of arsenic. Besides it's just one of dozens of ingredients you can use as a base powder. Other excellent base powder choices to use alone or in combination include:

- corn flour
- corn starch
- rice flour
- French clay
- powdered calendula flowers
- powdered chamomile flowers

My favorite mixture is one part corn starch, one part arrowroot, and one part powdered calendula flowers. This mixture makes for a very light powder. Sometimes I just use 100% corn starch.

To the base powder, add your favorite essential oil. There you have it — a delightful, all-natural body powder!

GIFT IDEA

Herbal body powders make great Christmas stocking stuffers, Mother's Day, Valentine's Day, or baby shower gifts. Make one of the following recipes and divide it in half or thirds. Find a decorative tin or small powder box that you've stenciled with an ivy or floral design, add the herbal powder so that it fills two-thirds of the container, and add a satin puff or small, fuzzy, fluff brush inside. Top with a bow and label. Some craft stores carry shaker containers, which are always nice for storing body powder. Each recipe will make two to three gifts.

LAVENDER POWDER

¾ pound (340 g) base
powder mixture
½ pound (227 g) powdered
lavender flowers
1 to 4 ounces (28 to 112 g)
powdered rose
buds/petals (optional)
1 ounce (28 g) powdered
benzoin gum
½ ounce (14 g) essential oil
of lavender or rose
geranium (may mix
50/50 — makes a nice
floral fragrance)

Good for: all skin types
Use: as desired
Prep time: 3 days
Mix with: mortar and pestle, flour sifter or food processor, spoon
Store in: zip-seal bag, box, tin, plastic tub, or shaker container
Yields: approximately 24 ounces
Special: Makes a light, lovely, old-fashioned floral-scented body powder.

Combine ingredients in a large bowl or food processor, except the essential oil. Stir with a large spoon or whiz in the food processor for 30 seconds until well blended. Using a mortar and pestle, combine the oil with a few tablespoons of powder until oil is absorbed. Add this mixture to remaining powder and sift together or shake vigorously in a large container with a tight-fitting lid. Whiz for 30 seconds, again, if using a food processor. Store powder in an airtight container and put in a cool, dark place for about 3 days so that the oil can permeate the powder. Use as you would any body powder.

This recipe makes a rather large amount of powder. You may store a portion of the powder in a decorative container for your present use, and the remainder in any airtight container, in a cool, dark place for future use.

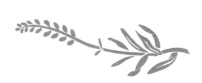

SANDALWOOD POWDER

1 pound (454 g) base pow-
der mixture
1 vanilla bean, chopped into
½ -inch pieces
1 ounce (28 g) powdered
benzoin gum
½ ounce (14 g) essential oil
of sandalwood

Good for: all skin types
Use: as desired
Prep time: 3 days
Mix with: mortar and pestle, flour sifter
or food processor, spoon
Store in: zip-seal bag, box, tin, plastic
tub, or shaker container
Yields: approximately 17 ounces (476 g)
Special: Has an earthy, sensual fragrance.

Combine ingredients in a large bowl or food processor, except the essential oil. Stir with a large spoon or whiz in the food processor for 30 seconds until well blended. Using a mortar and pestle, combine the oil with a few tablespoons of powder until oil is absorbed. Add this mixture to remaining powder and sift together or shake vigorously in a large container with a tight-fitting lid. Whiz for 30 seconds, again, if using a food processor. Store powder in an airtight container and put in a cool, dark place for about 3 days so that the oil can permeate the powder. Use as you would any body powder.

You may leave the vanilla bean pieces in the powder if you wish, or simply remove and save them for other uses.

BABY POWDER

½ pound (227 g) base pow-
der mixture
½ pound (227 g) powdered
chamomile, calendula
(pot marigold), or elder
flowers

Good for: all skin types, especially sensitive and delicate baby's skin
Use: as desired
Prep time: 10 to 15 minutes
Mix with: large bowl and spoon or food
processor
Store in: zip-seal bag, box, tin, plastic
tub, or shaker container
Yields: approximately 16 ounces (454 g)
Special: Has a very faint, delicate scent. It
is a light, soothing, all-purpose powder.

Mix ingredients thoroughly in a large bowl or food processor. Store.

REFRESHING FOOT POWDER

½ pound (227 g) powder
   base mixture
¼ pound (113 g) powdered
   peppermint
15 drops each essential oil
   of peppermint, eucalyptus, and cajeput
½ ounce (14 g) powdered
   benzoin gum

Good for: all skin types, and especially tired, smelly feet

Use: as desired

Prep time: 3 days

Mix with: mortar and pestle, flour sifter or food processor, spoon

Store in: zip-seal bag, box, tin, plastic tub, or shaker container

Yields: approximately 12 ounces (336 g)

Special: This powder is also nice to use during and after exercise, especially in hot weather.

Combine ingredients in a large bowl or food processor, except the essential oil. Stir with a large spoon or whiz in the food processor for 30 seconds until well blended. Using a mortar and pestle, combine the oil with a few tablespoons of powder until oil is absorbed. Add this mixture to remaining powder and sift together or shake vigorously in a large container with a tight-fitting lid. Whiz for 30 seconds, again, if using a food processor. Store powder in an airtight container and put in a cool, dark place for about 3 days so that the oil can permeate the powder. Use as you would any body powder.

This powder should be sprinkled on clean, dry feet prior to exercise so as to ease friction between toes and shoes and to absorb sweat.

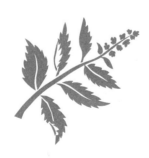

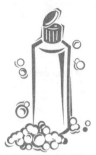

SHAMPOOS, RINSES, AND CONDITIONERS

Most men and women today style their hair to some degree daily. Whether it's simply a quick blow-dry or a complex ritual of moussing, blow-drying, using hot rollers, brushing, applying gel, then topping it all off with hair spray, your hair takes a lot of abuse. There's another factor to consider too . . . environmental stress. Sunshine, salt water, chlorine, smoking, pollution, and dry office air, all take their toll on your hair's health. Some of you, myself included, have a simple wash-and-wear style, but have a tendency to shampoo quite often, which can strip away your hair's natural oils and leave your crowning glory like straw.

Hair is not meant to take this kind of constant torture. Do your best to find a hair stylist who will cut your hair in a style that it naturally falls into with minimal effort. This will cut down on the number of harsh styling aids you need, shorten your styling time, and it just might save your hair.

GIFT IDEA

Herbal shampoos and conditioners make nice gifts for a special friend.

These recipes can be given in glass or plastic bottles, labeled with instructions, and "wrapped" in a decorative wine bag or gift bag. If you want to give a bottle of Highlight Booster, be sure to tell your friend to refrigerate it. The only recipes I wouldn't give as gifts are the dandruff treatment formulations — unless you and your friend are very close!

If you feel as if you can't live without spray or gels, try your local health food store. There are several natural, nontoxic brands now on the market, and many come in recyclable containers.

The following recipes are quite simple to make and with consistent use will improve the condition of your hair and scalp. The rosemary, chamomile, and calendula rinse recipes will give your highlights a color boost as well as leave your hair very soft and shiny.

HAIR CONDITIONER AND SCALP STIMULATOR

1 teaspoon (5 ml) essential oil of lemongrass

5 teaspoons (25 ml) essential oil of rosemary

3 teaspoons (15 ml) essential oil of lavender

4 teaspoons (20 ml) essential oil of basil

2 teaspoons (10 ml) essential oil of lemon

2 teaspoons (10 ml) essential oil of sandalwood

10 teaspoons (50 ml) jojoba oil

Good for: all hair types
Use: daily or as desired
Follow with: shampoo
Prep time: 5 to 10 minutes
Mix with: shake before use
Store in: dark bottle with dropper or any small, dark, glass bottle
Yields: approximately 14 treatments
Special: Helps stimulate circulation and remove dandruff buildup.

Combine oils and keep tightly closed, in a cool, dark place. Massage 2 teaspoons (10 ml) into your dry scalp for about 2 to 3 minutes and rub a little onto the ends of your hair. You're not trying to cover your entire head, just the scalp and ends. Wrap your head in plastic or use a shower cap, then wrap again with a very warm, damp towel. Leave on 30 to 45 minutes. Rinse and shampoo.

This conditioner can also be applied in the shower to a warm, wet scalp. Massage, allow to remain in your hair about 3 minutes or longer, rinse, and shampoo. This mixture has a strong fragrance and may tingle slightly — quite invigorating!

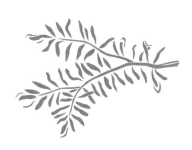

BASIC OIL CONDITIONER

¼ cup (60 ml) more or less (depending on length of hair) of one of the following oils: virgin olive, jojoba, sweet almond, or castor

10 drops essential oil of lavender, rosemary, or basil

Good for: normal and dry hair
Use: one time per week
Follow with: shampoo
Prep time: approximately 1 minute
Yields: 1 treatment
Special: Excellent for dry, sun-damaged, and chemically treated hair. Leaves hair soft and silky.

Combine the oils and apply to warm, damp (not wet) clean hair. Make sure hair is thoroughly coated. Cover with a plastic bag or shower cap, then cover again with a hot, damp towel. The heat helps the oil to penetrate and condition your hair. Allow to remain on for 30 minutes, then shampoo twice to remove all traces of oil.

FRAGRANT HAIR SHEEN

Essential oil of rosemary, lavender, or sandalwood

Good for: normal and dry hair
Use: after every shampoo or as desired
Special: Makes hair fragrant and shiny.

In the palm of your hand, place 5 drops essential oil of your choice or 2 drops of each of the oils. Rub palms together and gently pat and scrunch your slightly damp hair. Make sure to distribute oils evenly, paying special attention to ends.

If you set your hair, apply immediately before setting. If you use a blow dryer, apply in the middle of the styling process.

HERBAL SHAMPOO FOR ALL HAIR TYPES

2 cups (500 ml) distilled water

1 tablespoon (15 ml) calendula (pot marigold)

2 teaspoons (10 ml) rosemary

1 tablespoon (15 ml) nettle

2 teaspoons (10 ml) orange peel

2 teaspoons (10 ml) comfrey

2 tablespoons (30 ml) chamomile

½ teaspoon (2.5 ml) essential oil of lavender

1 teaspoon (5 ml) jojoba oil (omit if hair is oily)

½ cup (125 ml) all-natural, gentle baby shampoo

Good for: all hair types

Use: daily or as needed

Follow with: your regular conditioner, Basic Oil Conditioner, Hair Sheen, or Highlight Booster

Prep time: approximately 45 minutes

Mix with: medium-sized bowl and spoon

Store in: bottle

Yields: approximately 40 treatments

Special: Leaves hair shiny and soft. Good baby shampoo, very mild and gentle.

Bring water to a boil and remove from heat. Add the herbs, cover, and allow to steep for 30 minutes. Strain mixture into a medium-sized bowl, add the oils and stir vigorously. Add the shampoo and gently stir until thoroughly mixed. Pour into a labeled bottle and keep refrigerated to preserve the freshness. You may keep a small bottle in the shower with enough shampoo for about one week, if you wish. Use approximately 1 tablespoon (15 ml) per application. This shampoo will not produce mountains of billowy suds as it does not contain strong foaming agents. It cleans gently with minimal sudsing.

   Note: Before use, lightly shake shampoo to mix the oil that may separate from the rest of the ingredients.

HERBAL SHAMPOO FOR OILY HAIR

2 cups (500 ml) distilled
water

1 tablespoon (15 ml) bur-
dock seeds (crushed)
or leaves

1 tablespoon (15 ml) pep-
permint

1 tablespoon (15 ml) lemon
grass

1 tablespoon (15 ml) yarrow

¼ teaspoon (1.25 ml)
essential oil of clary
sage, tea tree, or rose-
mary

½ cup (125 ml) all-natural,
baby shampoo

Good for: oily hair

Use: daily or as needed

Follow with: your regular conditioner or Highlight Booster

Prep time: approximately 45 minutes

Mix with: medium-sized bowl and spoon

Store in: bottle

Yields: approximately 40 treatments

Special: Leaves hair soft and shiny and in good condition. In a pinch, can double as a face wash.

Bring water to a boil and remove from heat. Add the herbs, cover, and allow to steep for 30 minutes. Strain mixture into a medium-sized bowl, add the oil and stir vigorously. Add the shampoo and gently stir until thoroughly mixed. Pour into a labeled bottle and keep refrigerated to preserve the freshness of the herbal liquid. You may keep a small bottle in the shower with enough shampoo for about a week, if you wish. Use approximately 1 tablespoon (15 ml) per application.

HIGHLIGHT BOOSTERS

3 cups (750 ml) distilled or spring water

Brown/black hair — sage, rosemary, quassia chips, crushed walnut hulls

Blonde hair — chamomile, crushed rhubarb root

Red hair — calendula (pot marigold)

Good for: Rosemary, chamomile, and calendula can be used on any type of hair. The other herbs are somewhat astringent, and best used on hair that is normal or oily. If necessary, follow the rinse with a leave-in conditioner to counteract the drying effect of these herbs.

Use: daily or as needed

Follow with: conditioner, if necessary

Prep time: 35 to 40 minutes

Mix with: spoon

Store in: bottle

Yields: 3 to 5 treatments

Bring water to a boil and remove from heat. Add 3 heaping tablespoons (45 to 50 ml) of the herb(s) of your choice, stir, cover, and allow to steep for 30 minutes. Strain, label, and store in a quart-sized plastic bottle. Keep refrigerated.

Shampoo hair, rinse. Squeeze out excess water from hair, then generously pour herbal liquid until hair is saturated. Squeeze out excess.

If you'd like to make a mild shampoo, cut your usual shampoo 50/50 with the rinse of your choice and shampoo as usual. Mild mixture does not need to be refrigerated if used within two weeks.

Note: Use dark towels when drying hair as the herbal liquid will stain lighter-colored ones.

RINSE TO DARKEN GRAY HAIR

8 cups (2 liters) distilled
or spring water
1 ounce (28 g) sage
2 ounces (56 g) black
walnut hulls
2 tablespoons (30 ml)
regular loose tea (2
teabags will do fine)
1 ounce (28 g) rosemary
1 ounce (28 g) nettle
2 teaspoons (10 ml) jojoba,
castor, sweet almond,
or virgin olive oil
rubber or latex gloves

Good for: medium-to-dark gray, light-to-dark brown and auburn hair; for all hair types except very dry and/or chemically treated

Use: daily for 2 weeks, then as desired

Follow with: good quality conditioner

Prep time: approximately 4 hours

Mix with: shake before use

Store in: quart-sized bottles

Yields: approximately 16 treatments

Special: Leaves hair shiny and soft.

Boil water and remove from heat. Add herbs, cover, and steep for 3 to 4 hours. Strain, add oil, and store in refrigerator. Discard any remaining liquid after 3 weeks. Shampoo as usual and rinse. Before you begin this procedure, put on your gloves. This rinse will stain hands and nails dark brown. Shake bottle thoroughly, and apply about ½ cup (125 ml) of the herbal liquid and massage into scalp and hair for about 1 minute. Squeeze out excess and towel dry hair. Make sure you use a dark towel as this mixture *will stain* lighter-colored ones.

I usually get on my knees and hang my head over the bath tub when I do this rinse. If it splatters in the tub or on your face, it will wipe off.

I also wash my hair using 1 tablespoon (15 ml) of a mixture of ¼ cup (60 ml) baby shampoo and ¼ cup (60 ml) of this dark rinse. No gloves necessary for this treatment. I use it daily and doctor it with ¼ teaspoon (1.25 ml) each essential oil of lavender and rosemary and a few drops of jojoba oil. Discard this mixture after 2 weeks.

Note: The more porous your hair, the more quickly the hair strands will absorb the color. Thick, coarse hair will be quite resistant to taking any herbal color. Everyone's hair is different. Some gray may turn light brown, dark blonde, or medium-to-dark brown.

Anti-Dandruff Treatments

If you begin to see those pesky white flakes in your hair or on your shoulders, it's best to avoid or at least minimize the use of hair gels and sprays, hot blow dryers, harsh shampoos, perms, colors, and straighteners. These can cause a flaky, dry scalp which can imitate dandruff. True dandruff itches and can be a result of hormonal disturbances, faulty diet, emotional stress, or an infection. For a very stubborn case of dandruff, consult your physician; otherwise, the recipes below work quite well.

ROSEMARY SOFTENING RINSE

4 cups (1000 ml) distilled
   or spring water
½ cup (125 ml) rosemary
1 teaspoon (5 ml) borax

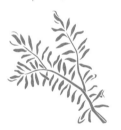

Good for: all hair types, especially lifeless, dull, and flaky
Use: daily or as desired
Follow with: Fragrant Hair Sheen, if desired
Prep time: approximately 2 hours
Mix with: spoon
Store in: bottle
Yields: 4 to 8 rinses, depending on length of hair
Special: Gives hair lustre and body.

Bring water to a boil and remove from heat. Add herbs and borax, stir, cover, and steep for approximately 2 hours. Strain, bottle, and use within 10 days or discard. Use as the final rinse after shampooing and conditioning. Do not rinse out. May stain light-colored towels. Use approximately ½ to 1 cup (125 to 250 ml) per application.

HERBAL VINEGAR INFUSION

2 cups (500 ml) distilled
  or spring water
½ cup (125 ml) apple cider
  vinegar
4 tablespoons (60 ml)
  rosemary
1 tablespoon (15 ml) nettle
10 drops essential oil of
  tea tree, clary sage, or
  rosemary

Good for: all hair types, except very dry
Use: daily or as needed
Follow with: Fragrant Hair Sheen, if
desired, or leave-in conditioner
Prep time: approximately 2 hours
Mix with: shake before use
Store in: bottle
Yields: approximately 10 treatments
Special: Helps to relieve an itchy scalp
and restores pH balance.

Bring the water and vinegar to a boil. Remove from heat. Add herbs, cover, and steep for about 2 hours. Strain, add essential oil, and bottle. No need to refrigerate. Shampoo hair and rinse, or, if not shampooing, wet hair and squeeze out excess. Apply approximately ¼ cup (60 ml) to wet scalp and gently massage for 2 to 3 minutes. Rinse with cool water. Try to use daily until itching and flaking stops.

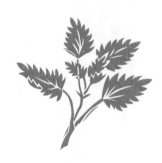

DENTIFRICES AND MOUTHWASHES

Most commercial toothpastes on the market today contain harsh abrasives, which, over the years, wear down tooth enamel and gum tissue. Many also contain saccharin, sugar, and detergents. Most mouthwashes aren't any better. They're colored with artificial dyes and flavor, contain alcohol, and harsh chemicals. Why submit your teeth and gums to such torture? Try a gentle, natural approach by using the following recipes.

Note: If you have chronic bad breath or dental problems, see your dentist.

GIFT IDEA

To give a lovely basket of just dental hygiene products is like saying, in a not-so-subtle way, "Gee, your breath smells horrible . . . but I hope you have a nice day, anyway." This is not advisable! It would be better to give a "sampler basket." By this I mean, combine a body powder and massage oil with a hand cream and an herbal mouthwash. This way your friend can sample the variety of herbal products you make, without being offended.

ANTISEPTIC MOUTHWASH AND GARGLE

6 ounces (180 ml) of
   water
3 to 4 drops essential oil
   of clove or tea tree

Good for: sore, bleeding gums, cold sores in the mouth, and sore throat
Use: daily or as needed
Prep time: approximately 1 minute
Mix with: spoon
Store in: Do not store. Mix as needed.
Yields: 1 treatment
Special: Mouth should feel cool and possibly a bit numb.

Stir water and oil together in a small glass. Swish in your mouth and gargle for 30 seconds, then spit out. Repeat 1 to 2 more times. May use this mixture throughout the day to help relieve sore throat and cold sores if necessary.

SODA/SALT PASTE

1 teaspoon (5 ml) baking soda or finely ground sea salt
1 drop essential oil of peppermint, clove, cinnamon, or spearmint
Few drops of water

Good for: everyone
Use: daily
Follow with: water rinse or mouthwash
Prep time: 1 to 2 minutes
Mix with: toothbrush and small bowl
Store in: Do not store. Mix as needed.
Yields: 1 treatment
Special: Leaves mouth feeling clean and fresh. Cinnamon oil may irritate sensitive gums and tongue.

Combine ingredients in a tiny bowl and mix thoroughly until a smooth, thick paste forms. Don't make it too runny or it won't stay on your toothbrush. Use as you would your regular toothpaste.

STRAWBERRY BRIGHTENER

1 medium-sized ripe strawberry

Good for: everyone, especially those with stained teeth
Use: daily
Follow with: water rinse or mouthwash
Prep time: approximately 1 minute
Mix with: mash fruit with mortar and pestle
Yields: 1 treatment
Special: Leaves mouth feeling clean and wonderful tasting.

Mash strawberry into a pulp. Dip your brush into the liquid and brush normally. Strawberries have a slight bleaching effect and help to rid the teeth of tea, coffee, and cigarette stains. A strawberry is much safer to use than lemon juice, which is too acidic.

TOOTH TWIG

3-inch to 4-inch twig from a sweet gum or flowering dogwood tree (twig must be "just cut" from the tree)

Good for: everyone
Use: daily
Follow with: water rinse or mouthwash
Prep time: 2 to 3 minutes
Yields: 1 treatment
Special: This is definitely a recyclable toothbrush, about as natural as they come!

Peel the twig and chew on the end until it is frayed and soft. It should taste slightly sweet. Now gently rub your teeth and gums. This is a very "old fashioned" way of brushing your teeth, but it's effective. The twig can also be dipped in water and baking soda, if you desire.

HERBAL MOUTHWASH

2 cups (500 ml) distilled water
2 tablespoons (30 ml) peppermint, spearmint, or rosemary
10 drops tincture of benzoin or 1 teaspoon (5 ml) tincture of myrrh

Good for: everyone, especially those with bad breath, sore and/or bleeding gums
Use: daily
Prep time: approximately 8 hours or overnight
Mix with: shake before use
Store in: bottle
Yields: approximately 16 rinses
Special: Leaves mouth feeling cool and tingly.

Boil water and remove from heat. Add herb of choice, cover, and steep for about 8 hours or overnight. After the liquid has cooled, you can put the pot in the refrigerator to steep overnight, if you wish. Strain, add either tincture (acts as a preservative and antiseptic), and bottle. Use approximately 2 tablespoons (30 ml) per use.

SUNSCREEN

Light to moderate exposure to the sun makes us feel good; helps the body manufacture vitamin D; gives us energy after a long, cold winter; warms the soul; and leaves a rosy-golden glow upon the skin. On the flipside, overexposure dries our skin; causes wrinkles, blotchiness, and premature aging; and, increasingly, leads to skin cancer. If you are going to be in the sun for a period of time, by all means apply a good sunscreen. This is especially important if you're going to be on or near water, or even relaxing on a sandy beach. Water and sand can reflect the sun's powerful rays, further increasing the chances of overexposure and skin damage.

SUNSCREEN BODY OIL

¼ cup (60 ml) anhydrous lanolin

¼ cup (60 ml) light sesame oil

4 teaspoons (20 ml) vitamin E oil

¼ cup (60 ml) sweet almond oil

⅓ cup (80 ml) aloe vera gel

15 drops essential oil of sandalwood or bitter almond

Good for: normal and dry skin; dark or tanned skin or when *minimal* sunscreen protection is desired

Use: before and during sun exposure

Prep time: approximately 10 minutes

Mix with: shake before use

Store in: plastic squeeze bottle

Yields: approximately 9 applications

Special: Makes a great after-bath skin softener.

Combine all ingredients in one or two squeeze bottles. Store the bottle you're not using in the refrigerator. Use approximately 2 tablespoons (30 ml) per use. Use unrefrigerated oil within 3 weeks or discard.

SUNBURN RELIEF SUGGESTIONS

1. Add 2 cups (500 ml) apple cider vinegar to cool bath water and soak for 10 to 20 minutes.
2. Apply cold aloe vera gel directly to sunburn. Apply several times per day.
3. Apply cold, strong, regular tea directly to sunburn with soaked cotton pads. Apply several times per day.

FOR WOMEN ONLY: DOUCHES

Most dry form and premixed douches are chemical-based and can strip the natural protective pH of the vagina. As an alternative, the following recipes are very gentle. Keep in mind that these douches are not intended as a medical treatment but rather a cosmetic one. See your doctor if symptoms persist.

If you have any allergies related to plants, be sure to perform the patch test as described on page 9 before using either of these recipes.

VAGINITIS RELIEF

2 quarts (2 litres) luke-
warm water
¼ cup (60 ml) apple cider
vinegar **or** 10 drops
essential oil of tea tree

Good for: external itching and burning; cleans excess vaginal discharge
Use: one to two times per week. Do not use more often than this.
Prep time: approximately 2 minutes
Yields: 1 treatment
Special: Leaves a clean, fresh feeling.

Combine ingredients in a 2-quart (2 litres) douche bag and proceed as usual. See your doctor if symptoms persist.

FRESHENING DOUCHE

2 quarts (2 litres) water
2 tablespoons (30 ml)
peppermint, rosemary,
or yarrow

Good for: general cleansing and freshening
Use: one time per week
Prep time: approximately 2 hours
Yields: 1 treatment

Boil water and remove from heat. Add herb, cover, and steep for about 2 hours. Strain and pour into douche bag. Proceed as usual.

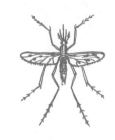

INSECT REPELLENT

This insect repellent recipe is a natural alternative to chemical sprays. It works best on days when the mosquitoes are only slightly to moderately hungry. If they're voracious, a stronger concoction will have to be sought.

BUGS BE GONE

2 cups (500 ml) witch hazel
1½ teaspoons (7.5 ml) essential oil of citronella or lemongrass
1 tablespoon (15 ml) apple cider vinegar

Good for: all skin types
Use: as needed
Prep time: 3 to 5 minutes
Mix with: shake before use
Store in: spritzer
Yields: approximately 50 applications for entire body
Special: Has a light, fresh fragrance.

Combine all ingredients in a 16-ounce (500 ml) spray bottle or two 8-ounce (240 ml) bottles. Shake vigorously. Requires no refrigeration. Apply liberally as needed. Keep away from eyes, nose, and mouth.

PART II:
SOOTHING HAND CARE

Herbal Treatments
and Simple Techniques
for Healthy Hands and Nails

Norma Pasekoff Weinberg

INTRODUCTION

There are easy, natural things we can do to promote our health and the well-being of this planet. It all begins with having the confidence to accept responsibility as caretaker, the capacity to respect each and every voice, and the willingness to try the uncomplicated approach first and, if necessary, advance to the next level of care only as needed. In most cases, the earth has been a nurturing place for its inhabitants, and it seems logical to turn to plants and natural remedies as a first line of defense in helping our bodies deal with temporary malaise.

I attempt to bridge two worlds in this section: the world of Western allopathic medicine, which respects laboratory research and controlled medical studies, and the world of folk herbal medicine, which is tested by a wide range of geographic use and the span of time. These approaches are not antagonistic. Both seek to help the individual to maintain or regain essential health. The allopathic approach often focuses on suppressing overt symptoms of disease (which we typically request in doctor's offices) while the herbalist approach takes the slower route, trying to work with the underlying causes and assist the body in rebuilding natural defenses.

Next to the brain, the hand represents humankind's greatest asset. This anatomic marvel has enabled humans to excel over all other species. In reality, the human hand functions to a large degree as an extension of the individual's brain. Witness the truly remarkable capacity of Helen Keller, who was both deaf and blind, to fulfill a meaningful life through her hands.

When humans became bipedal, our hands were relieved of the duty of locomotion and freed to develop into extremely useful and sophisticated instruments. The structures involved in tactile function are highly refined, and the machinery of the hand involves specialized tissues of great delicacy and sophistication. Witness the human thumb, unique in its strength, mobility, and size relative to the digits. With this highly evolved component, our hands have proven successful not only in fundamental tasks of survival but also in drawing, sculpting, and all of the precise, beautiful things that surround civilization.

This section will appeal to a wide audience of both professional and lay readers. Technical terms are minimized and the thrust of the section is away from the specialized issues of hand anatomy, function, and pathology. Rather, the section explores a wide range of issues related to both how the hand functions as well as the care of its component parts. It is sprinkled with vignettes bringing to the reader historical as well as contemporary issues as diverse as the history of nail polish to the life span of a wart. It is easy to read, accurate, and — of particular importance — useful.

After reading this text, few if any will ever take their hands for granted. From the perspective of a physician involved in the care of hand problems and traumatic disruptions of the hand, I was enthralled by this text, learned quite a few useful facts, and would recommend it equally to professionals involved in the care of the hand as well as to anyone who takes pride in their hands' appearance and function.

—Jesse B. Jupiter, M.D.
Director of Orthopaedic Hand Service
(Massachusetts General Hospital),
Associate Professor of Orthopaedic Surgery
(Harvard Medical School),
Editor, *Flynn's Hand Surgery,* 4th ed.
(Williams & Wilkins, 1990)

CHAPTER 3
Basic Steps to Beautiful Hands
▀▀▀▀▀

*Healing is simply attempting to do more of those things
that bring joy and fewer of those things that bring pain.*
— O. Carl Simonton, *The Healing Journey*

Our skin is the shield that protects the inner body from the stones and arrows of the outside environment. If you want a warranty from the manufacturer for long-term use, it's essential to find a natural routine that takes care of and maintains this protective equipment.

SUNBATHING IN THE NUDE

I knew that would get your attention! Nude sunbathing is what you do every time you venture out without covering your hands and arms with protective clothing or sunscreen. Depleting ozone layers dictate that you must protect the skin from the effects of ultraviolet radiation, both UVA and UVB — and if our ozone layer continues to be consumed, it will soon be UVC as well. Photoaging of the skin (rough, leathery texture, sagging skin, and brown-pigmented, freckle-like spots on the backs of the hands) is caused by undue exposure to sunlight.

Here's how. Long-term sun exposure degrades the skin's support network of collagen and elastin fibers and causes the skin to become less flexible. Research also points to other possible problems with excess sunbathing that include precancerous or cancerous growths due to changes in the body's DNA codes, and the possibility of a compromised immune response due to destruction of certain white blood cells (the helper T-cells). Each individual is different, and so is tolerance to sun exposure. Every one of us deserves some sunshine in our lives, but for beautiful, healthy skin, moderation is the key. If you're going to be outdoors for any length of time, wear sunscreen. It will protect your skin against sunburn and premature wrinkles. And don't forget to apply sunscreen to your hands.

SEVEN BASIC STEPS TO HEALTHY HANDS

1. Eat right. Choose foods as close to the way they were "born" as possible. Vary the types of fruits and vegetables.
2. Drink at least 6 glasses of pure water a day to keep the skin moisturized inside and out.
3. Get the sleep your body needs.
4. Wear sunscreen or protective clothing to avoid overexposing that "baby" skin to the elements. Some sunshine is necessary for the body and soul. However, today's suntan is tomorrow's aging skin.
5. Wash with mild cleansers. Avoid temperature extremes and harsh detergents. As a normal skin function, sweat and sebaceous glands routinely rid the body of toxins and wastes.
6. Protect your hands with moisturizing creams, sunscreen, or the appropriate gloves when you are exposing your hands to abrasive or outside elements.
7. Exercise. When you are faced with repetitive tasks, take time out to stretch and wiggle your fingers, wrists, hands, and arms to maintain normal range of movement.

GLOVES FOR EVERY REASON

Human skin comes wrapped and sealed with its own natural skin cream made of sebum, lecithin, cholesterol, and water. We do our best to break down this natural environmental barrier using hot water, detergents, solvents, polishes, and waxes that dehydrate the skin and remove its natural protective oils. Need an example? We have such a compulsion to keep things clean and shiny that it is difficult to keep our naked hands out of hot water. This behavior often results in "dishpan hands" and yeast infections around the nails. In solving this dilemma, it's gloves to the rescue. Whether you are washing, cleaning, or otherwise handling harsh materials, wear gloves to protect your hands against the elements.

Fabrics for gloves have come a long way from the days of metal chains, linen, and silk. Today gloves and mittens are made from every material you can think of, including canvas, cotton, nylon, terry cloth, wool, cowhide, deerskin, goatskin, latex, pigskin, polypropylene, rubber, suede, split leather, and vinyl.

Gloves are also available in every color of the rainbow and more. There are camouflage gloves for sportsmen; garden gloves with floral prints; water-repellent gloves with cotton-knit lining in colors coordinated to match any kitchen; and fluorescent, neon gloves with foam insulation and fleece lining ideal for shoveling snow while also making the occasional lost glove visible in a snowy yard.

IF THE GLOVE FITS, WEAR IT

There are varieties of gloves available today for every purpose you can imagine, and even for some you never imagined. In many cases, each glove is designed and manufactured to protect the hand against a particular environmental, chemical, or skin-destructive condition.

THROW DOWN THE GAUNTLET

Gloves have probably been worn since Adam left the cozy Garden of Eden. The earliest remnants of gloves have been found in Egypt, in the tomb of the pharaoh Tutankhamen, dating about 1350 B.C.E. In the Middle Ages, knights used gloves both as a challenge to combat and as a pledge of honor. Throwing a glove on the ground to be picked up by the person being challenged was the way a duel was arranged. In Scotland, "to bite a glove" was considered a pledge of vengeance that could be ended only by death.

At jousts during this age of chivalry, the glove was a love token a lady presented to her knight to be worn on his helmet during battle. Gloves in those days were handmade of linen, silk, velvet, or kid and were highly ornamented. Knights in armor protected their own hands with fingerless gloves, strengthened by chain mail or metal plates.

It wasn't until 1834 that gloves became available to regular folks not endowed with the riches of nobles, bishops, emperors, or queens. In that year, Xavier Jouvin, a glovemaker in Grenoble, France, invented the punch press, which simultaneously cut out six gloves and so spawned mass production. Not long afterward, in 1845, the invention of the sewing machine completely revolutionized glove making. Cotton and synthetic materials also helped to put gloves in the price range and reach of the general population.

Glove Tips for Gardening and Wet Work

Gloves are particularly useful for gardening and working in wet or cold conditions. They'll protect your hands from irritants such as fertilizers and pesticides and keep the skin from becoming raw and chapped. (Garden glove tips come courtesy of horticulturists Bruce Roberts and Suzanne Siegel of the Massachusetts Horticultural Society.)

◆ Always wear gloves when you have to do wet work.

◆ Cotton gloves do not provide adequate hand protection when working with plant pesticides or other chemicals. It's wiser to use lined, industrial-grade, rubber-type gloves for these applications. Recheck gloves for splits before each use and toss those that don't meet specs.

◆ Dark brown, cotton knit jersey gloves, available in various densities, are just right for working with tender plant material, especially for transplanting seedlings. You'll find them comfortable, durable, and washable.

◆ High-cuff leather gloves are what you need to protect your hands when pruning roses, shrubs, and trees.

◆ Choose gloves with a natural fiber lining to protect hands against possible allergic reactions.

◆ Make sure the gloves are long enough so that water or chemicals will not splash inside when you are engaged in messy work.

◆ Try not to wear gloves for wet work for more than one hour at a time.

◆ If you do have a skin condition such as eczema on your hands, be sure to turn your gloves inside out several times a week and wash them.

◆ Inspect gloves daily, prior to wearing, to ensure that there are no holes or tears to either the inside or the outside surface.

◆ Discard torn gloves.

NATURAL HAND CLEANSERS
AND MOISTURIZERS

Washing your hands often is one of the best ways to stop the spread of germs and remove harmful atmospheric pollutants. Choose mild, natural ingredients for your hand cleansers, and apply barrier creams after cleansing to preserve the skin's moisture. This may surprise you, but pure water is one of the best ways to cleanse the skin. Water will remove soluble environmental pollutants such as compounds of sulfur and nitrogen, metal salts, and other chemicals, and with a neutral pH of 7.0, water accomplishes all this without disturbing the natural acid mantle of the skin.

Normal skin has a pH factor of 4.0 to 6.0. Tests show that skin with a normal pH of 4.0 rises to a pH of 7.0 one minute after washing with soap. If cider vinegar, which has a pH between 3.0 and 4.0, is applied to the skin after bathing, the pH factor will return to its normal range. However, the secret with skin-care products is to look for those that use natural ingredients. Avoid harsh, synthetic chemicals.

Natural and Herbal Hand Cleansers

Milk, sour milk, cream (used by Cleopatra, it is said), and buttermilk are all gentle skin cleansers. The next time you're in the kitchen, try washing with ¼ cup (60 ml) of fresh or sour milk, buttermilk, or cream instead of one of the liquid dish detergents. It is a surprisingly pleasant experience.

To remove greasy substances not removed by water or milk, try an exfoliant such as cornmeal or oatmeal. A heavy hand is not needed. The grainy texture releases both dirt and dead surface skin while stimulating the new skin cells below. Or try the Grainy Hands Soap Substitute recipe on page 83 or the Special Wash for Chapped Hands on page 135.

GRAINY HANDS SOAP SUBSTITUTE

Make a batch to have "on hand."

1 cup (250 ml) cornmeal or oatmeal, finely ground

2 cups (500 ml) white kaolin clay, finely powdered

1/4 cup (60 ml) almonds, finely ground (leave just a bit of grittiness)

1/4 cup (60 ml) dried lavender blossoms, finely powdered

1/8 cup (30 ml) dried rose petals, finely powdered

A few drops of the essential oil of your choice (optional)

A pinch of dried kelp (optional)

A pinch of powdered vitamin C (optional)

Liquid contents of a 400 IU vitamin E capsule (optional)

To make:

Stir all ingredients together in a bowl and pour into a large jar. Store jar in a dry, cool location.

To use:

1. Mix 1 to 2 teaspoons (5–10 ml) of the cleansing grains with water.

2. Stir into a paste by rubbing your hands in a circular motion. Then work the grains up each individual finger and over the back of the hand.

3. Rinse with cool or lukewarm water. Pat dry.

Caution: This recipe may irritate sensitive skin.

(Adapted from a recipe by master herbalist Rosemary Gladstar.)

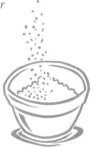

GRAINY HANDS SOAP SUBSTITUTE FOR CHAPPED HANDS

This is a variation of the Grainy Hands recipe for people whose hands are raw or chapped. Make small batches on an as-needed basis.

1–2 teaspoons (5–10 ml) Grainy Hands Soap Substitute (see page 83)

1 scant teaspoon (5 ml) honey

Distilled rose water

To make:

Add honey to the Grainy Hands Soap Substitute and enough rose water to make a paste.

To use:

1. Stir into a paste by rubbing your hands in a circular motion. Then work the grains up each individual finger and over the back of the hand.

2. Rinse with cool or lukewarm water. Pat dry.

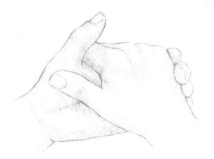

Natural and Herbal Hand Creams

If you want smoother, more pliable skin, get in the habit of using protective hand and nail creams. These creams help the skin retain moisture by adding to the natural, water-resistant (lipid) barrier between you and the environment. Soaps and detergents constantly erode this barrier. When applied to slightly damp skin, emollient creams, lotions, and ointments slow evaporation and hold on to vital moisture.

Which moisturizers are the best? The choice is yours. You might decide that at work you want a hand emollient that dries quickly and has no fragrance, has an oil-in-water (O/W) base, and is a lotion formula. At home you may use a water-in-oil (W/O) base, a cream formula, and one that you can wear all night with cotton gloves.

FROM THE FARM

Hand salves and creams have probably been around since the first peoples discovered bear grease. Many nineteenth-century hand products from the agricultural farm communities came with names like Absorbine Veterinary Liniment, Bag Balm, Corn Huskers Lotion, Thayer's Medicated Superhazel, and White Cloverine Salve. Farmers began to try these products, on the theory that "what's good for the horse is good for his owner."

One product, B and O'R Hand Lotion, conceived and produced by Vermont pharmacists Beauchamp and O'Rourke, was devised to cope with the industrial revolution. It was intended to protect ironworkers' hands from the temperature extremes of blast furnaces and the bitter Vermont cold. Witch hazel, camphor, soap liniment, glycerin, bay rum, rose water, and mutton tallow are some of the ingredients. It is still manufactured and sold today.

KITCHEN CABINET HAND LOTION

2 teaspoons (10 ml)
cod-liver oil

2 tablespoons (30 ml)
castor oil

2 soy lecithin capsules,
pierced and squeezed

1 natural vitamin E cap-
sule, pierced and
squeezed

1 tablespoon (15 ml)
unflavored gelatin

¼ cup (60 ml) cold water

¾ cup (180 ml) boiling
water

*(Adapted from a recipe by
Charles Dickson and
Ariel Mars.)*

To make:

1. In a blender, combine the cod-liver oil, castor oil, contents of the lecithin capsules, and contents of the vitamin E capsule.

2. Prepare the gelatin by dissolving it in the cold water.

3. Add the boiling water to the gelatin mixture. Stir till dissolved and then cool to room temperature.

4. Add ½ cup (125 ml) of the gelatin mixture to the blender. Blend thoroughly and add only enough water to achieve the consistency of a lotion.

5. Pour into a bottle and store in the refrigerator.

To use:

Use for dry or chapped hands.

QUICK AND EASY HAND SMOOTHING LOTION

1 tablespoon (15 ml)
glycerin

1 tablespoon (15 ml) rose
water

1 tablespoon (15 ml) non-
distilled witch hazel
extract

3 tablespoons (45 ml)
honey

To make:

1. Blend and shake well.

2. Store in the refrigerator.

To use: Pour a small amount into the palm of your hands and gently massage into your hands and fingers.

PERFECT MOISTURIZING HAND CREAM

The proportions of this cream are about 1 part oil base to 1 part water, essential oils, and vitamins. In the oil base ingredients, the proportions should be approximately 2 parts liquid oil to 1 part solid oil. Tap water is not recommended in the water ingredient because it can sometimes introduce bacteria to your cream that results in the growth of mold. If using aloe vera, the cream will be more dense but very moisturizing.

Oil Base Ingredients
3/4 cup (180 ml) apricot oil and/or sweet almond oil
1/2 cup (125 ml) coconut oil and/or cocoa butter
1 teaspoon (5 ml) anhydrous lanolin
1/2 ounce (14 g) grated beeswax

Water, Essential Oils, and Vitamins
2/3 cup (160 ml) distilled water, rose water, or orange flower water
1/3 cup (80 ml) aloe vera gel
A few drops of the essential oil of your choice
Vitamins A and E (optional)

(Thanks to Rosemary Gladstar and Sage Mountain Herbs for sharing this recipe.)

To make:

1. Heat the oil base ingredients over low heat in a double boiler until the solid oils are melted. Stir gently to mix well.

2. Pour the oil mixture into a glass measuring cup and cool to room temperature. The mixture should become thick, creamy, semisolid, and cream-colored. When completely cooled, you are ready for the next step.

3. Place the water, aloe, essential oil, and vitamins in a blender. Turn blender on the highest speed. In a slow, thin drizzle, pour the oil base mixture into the center hole of the blender.

4. When most of the oil base mixture has been added and the cream resembles a butter-cream frosting (you may not need to use all of the oil base mixture), turn off the blender. Do not overbeat. The cream should be rich and thick and continue to thicken as it sets up.

5. Pour into cream jars, label, and store in a cool place.

An Everyday Warm-Up Stretch and Massage for Your Hands

We work our hands hard and rarely take the time to care properly for them. Here are some basic limbering exercises and easy massages to do each morning while you are still in bed. They will tone and stretch your hand and arm muscles, stimulate circulation, and limber up your joints for the day ahead.

Step 1: Stretch
Reach your arms over your head and stretch your whole body. Feel your spine elongate. Relax. Now, reach your arms out to the sides. Stretch your rib cage and breathe deeply in and out. Notice how your abdomen rises on the inhale and falls on the exhale.

Step 2: Backs-of-hands massage
Rub the palm of the left hand over the back of the right hand; repeat the action with the palm of the right hand rubbing the back of the left hand, as if washing the hands. This stimulates circulation and warms the hands.

Step 3: Finger milking
With your right hand, "milk" each finger and thumb on the left hand (as if you were milking a cow or a goat). Begin closer to your knuckles and gently but firmly pull, squeeze, and work your way down to the fingertips. Repeat on the opposite hand.

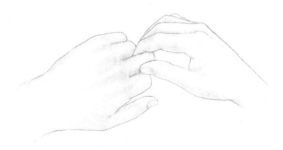

Step 4: Nail press

With the thumb and index finger of the opposite hand, press on each nail and do a gentle twist and rock, to bring circulation to the fingertips.

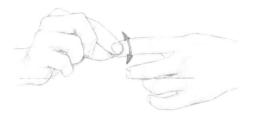

Step 5: Wrist circles

While lying on your back, form large, lazy circles with your arms, using your shoulders. Gradually work down to smaller and smaller circles until you are making just small, graceful circles with your wrists.

Step 6: Shake it out

It's time to sit up on the edge of the bed. With your arms hanging down by your sides, shake out both hands — first, loosely as a scarecrow, and then, rotating the thumb toward you and then away from you in a motion similar to the central post of a washing machine.

Step 7: Fists

Keeping your arms down, open and close your fists and squeeze your fingers into your palm (watch out for long nails!). This applies some pressure and encourages circulation.

Your hands are now ready to meet the day!

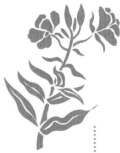

CHAPTER 4
Fingernail Diagnostics

Were it not for the fingers, the hand would be a spoon.

— African proverb

How many times during a day are your fingernails in use? Tell me about the itchy spot on your arm. Did you scratch it? And the dirty spot on the counter? Was it scraped away with the edge of a fingernail? Did you separate a sticky label from its backing or remove a staple with your nails? Our fingernails are truly our first tools. They help us manipulate fine objects and care for ourselves, and are a unique site for personal adornment.

In everyday life, our extremely "handy" fingernails are most conspicuous for how they decorate us. But whether fingernails receive credit for augmenting our appearance or for their convenience and service, it's worthwhile to know how to take care of them. Once you understand the basics, it will be easy to have and maintain healthy nails for the rest of your life.

WHAT MAKES A FINGERNAIL?

Probably the only time we focus on our fingernails is when we break or chip one and have to repair it. But nails offer us more than a fashion statement. Why do we have fingernails? A major responsibility of nails is shielding the delicate nerve endings at the tips of our fingers. Fingernails also contribute to the precision and sensation of touch, enhancing our dexterity and aiding the fingers in grasping objects. Our nails harbor the sensations of touch, temperature, and pain.

Nail Matrix

Nail growth begins in the nail matrix. Like human hair, the hard plate of fingernails is composed of a tough protein called keratin. Matrix cells make the keratin that becomes the visible, strong fingernail. The nail matrix, where the matrix cells collect, contains the nerves, lymph vessels, and blood vessels vital for nourishing the fingernails.

Nail Bed and Nail Plate

The nail bed is, appropriately enough, the bed of skin on which the nail plate and nail matrix rest. As keratin forms in the nail matrix, it pushes further forward onto the nail bed to harden and become the exposed nail plate (the clear shield commonly thought of as the fingernail). The tough nail plate contains none of the nerves or blood vessels found in the nail bed. It's no longer living tissue. Although the nail plate appears to be one solid piece, it is actually constructed in layers. You may notice these layers when a fingernail splits.

The record for having the world's longest nails is currently held by a woman in India. Picture fingernails that range in length from 40 to 52 inches (100 to 130 cm). That's 3 to 5 feet (90 to 150 cm) long! Imagine trying to take care of an itch!

For all they are able to do, it is surprising that normal nails are only 1/50 of an inch thick. When the nails are healthy, the nail plate remains firmly attached to the nail bed and continues to grow. Nail growth is dependent on good nutrition and general wellness.

Nail Fold

This layer of skin covers the edges of the nail plate on all sides except the tip, and holds the nail in place. It is often the primary site of nail fungus infections.

Cuticles

The cuticle, a small piece of skin that sometimes overhangs the nail plate, is one of the most important parts of the nail. The cuticle protects the nail matrix, the delicate tissues and cells below the nail plate that are actively forming the hard nail.

Any vigorous pushing back of the cuticles, trimming, or chemical solvents will cause ridges in the nail. And worse than ridges, once the cuticle is damaged, the watertight space under the nail fold is open to moisture and becomes a potential breeding ground for bacteria, yeast infections, and deformed nails.

Moons

We know that the birth of the fingernail takes place under the all-important cuticle. The milky white crescent formed at the base of the nail, crossed by the cuticle, is the half-moon, or lunula. This is a semi-transparent window to the nail matrix and nail bed underneath. The lunula is easiest to see on the thumb and hardest to see on the little finger. It may sometimes be obscured by the cuticle.

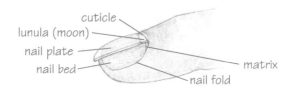

NAIL GROWTH

Fingernails wear down with use. Good biological planning arranged for nails to grow constantly during life. But there are variables that can affect how nails grow and nail growth, in turn, can offer information about your health and diet.

Following are some fingernail facts that you can use to impress your friends:

◆ Nail growth is different from person to person and from finger to finger. If your nails grow quickly, this is one measure that you are well nourished. Conversely, nails grow more slowly if you are ill or have a poor diet. In most cases, the nail on the middle finger grows the fastest and the nail on the little finger grows the slowest.

MOON SIGNS

It's been theorized that the size, shape, and color of fingernail "moons" are inherited. Compare the moons on your fingers to those of your family. Are they similar or different?

Lunulas that seem large for the nail may be an indication of an overactive thyroid gland. Not having moons on any of the nails may indicate an underactive thyroid gland or could be normal. Both of these "moon" conditions can be genetic and offer clues to a familial predisposition to certain health problems. Thyroid hormones stimulate the body's protein synthesis, oxygen consumption, and cell division and thereby affect the epidermis (the outer layer of skin). The effects of thyroid disease on the nails is still poorly understood, but the thyroid gland has a definite role in keratin production cycles of the hair and skin.

- As a rule, the nails of babies and older folks grow more slowly than those of teenagers.
- The length of the finger and the size of its moon suggest the speed of growth of the nail. The shorter the finger and the less of its visible moon, the more slowly the nail will grow. (The thumb is the exception.)
- Biting fingernails, while detrimental to their health in other ways, is thought to make them grow faster.
- Fingernails grow faster than toenails, and all nails grow more quickly in summer than in winter or cold weather. Heat increases the rate of all metabolic processes.
- Nails grow faster during the day than at night due to the natural pulse of body rhythms.
- Men's nails grow faster than women's. However, women will experience a spurt in nail growth just before menstruation and during pregnancy. These growth spurts are thought to be in response to hormonal activity.

NAIL NUTRITION

To keep fingernails healthy and strong, eat a healthy diet, including vitamin- and mineral-rich foods. Key vitamins and minerals for the nails are vitamins A, B-complex, C, D, E, iron, calcium, magnesium, zinc, sulfur, and essential fatty acids (EFA).

Remember, these elements, taken only as supplements, will be ineffective unless they are part of a varied, healthy diet. Nails grow slowly, so it will be at least three to four months into a fortified diet before you begin to see improvement in the quality of your nails.

FINGERNAIL DIAGNOSTICS

As early as 400 B.C.E., Hippocrates taught that the nails reflect the condition of the inner body. It is true that abnormalities of the nails can often provide early clues to common medical problems or severe systemic diseases.

We see color in the natural nail, but the fingernail itself is colorless and translucent. The central portion of the normal nail appears pink because the nail bed below the nail plate is rich in capillaries, and the nail plate is close-fitting. The free edge of the nail is white because of air beneath it. The lunula, or moon, appears white because it is not firmly attached to the nail plate.

But life can have an impact on our fingernails, changing their texture, hardness, color, thickness, and shape. These changes are worth noting because they speak to us of our inner health.

Lines and Ridges on the Fingernails

Take a few moments and examine your unpolished fingernails under a good light. You will gather a new appreciation for how your lifestyle affects your nails and overall health.

Long lines. As people age, longitudinal lines appear in the nails. These long lines are not considered important, and we know of no way to prevent them. Think of these lines as age wrinkles on the nails. (You'd have thought we would be safe from wrinkles somewhere on our bodies!)

There is some new thinking that long, corrugated lines on the nails may be due to the body's poor absorption of vitamins and minerals, or that these nail lines may signal anemia. More research is needed in this area. Some nutrients, in food and supplements, seem to be especially important in general nail health, including vitamins A, B-complex, and C, as well as calcium, magnesium, zinc, and essential fatty acids.

White lines. White lines across the nail bed are common, but sometimes are indications of liver or kidney disease.

Ridges. Any inflammation or irritation around the area of the nail matrix disturbs the growth pattern of the nail plate, and a lengthwise furrow is produced. Cuticle manipulation, such as cutting too much of the cuticle or pushing it back too vigorously, can cause fingernail ridging.

Beau's lines — horizontal ridges that cross the nail like wavy furrows — indicate that something has interrupted nail growth, such as high fever, nutritional deficiencies, drug reactions, painful menstruation, childbirth, or trauma from surgery. The nail matrix stops producing keratin. When the nail begins to grow again, a groove marks the spot where the nail-forming cells rested.

CLOCKING NAIL INJURIES

Nails grow at different rates due to age, nutrition, and health factors. Under the best of conditions, a nail grows about 0.004 inches (0.1 mm) a day or 1/8 of an inch (3 mm) each month. It takes about six months for a new nail to grow from cuticle to tip. If you're the scientific type, you can estimate the number of days since an illness or a trauma to the nail by measuring the distance from the horizontal ridge to the cuticle, or proximal nail fold. If the boo-boo occurred near the cuticle in January, it should be growing out by June.

Normal, healthy nails can grow in a variety of shapes, determined by a person's genetics. When we think about everyday fingernail problems, we most often focus on soft or brittle nails and split or pitted nails. These conditions are generally related to the effects of the environment, nail-biting, age, or heredity. However, changes in our nails can also be a signal of other internal health problems, and nail disorders can result from a variety of causes. The following chart outlines some common conditions to watch for.

NAIL DIAGNOSTICS

Nail Condition	Potential Cause
Complete loss of nail	Trauma to the nail; a form of dermatitis; syphilis
Nail plate loose	Injury; nail psoriasis; fungal or bacterial infections; medicines; chemotherapy; thyroid disease; Raynaud's phenomenon; lupus
Wasting away of nails; nail loses luster and becomes smaller	Injury or disease
Thickened nail plate	Poor circulation; fungal infection; heredity; mild, persistent trauma to the nail
Pitted nails sometimes with yellow-to-brown "oil" spots	Eczema or psoriasis; hair loss condition
Very soft nails	Contact with strong alkali; malnutrition; endocrine problems; chronic arthritis

Nail Condition	Potential Cause
Spoon-shaped nails	Iron deficiency; thyroid disease
Clublike nails growing around swollen finger ends	Chronic respiratory or heart problems; cirrhosis of the liver
Horizontal ridges	Injury; infection; nutrition
Longitudinal ridges	Aging; poor absorption of vitamins and minerals; thyroid disease; kidney failure
Brittle, split nails	Nail dryness; nails in contact with irritating substances (detergents, chemicals, polish remover); silica deficiency
Infected nails: red tender, swollen, pus	Bacterial or yeast infection
Overlarge moons	Overactive thyroid; genetics; self-induced trauma (habit tick)
No moons	Underactive thyroid; genetics

Discolored Fingernails

Normally, the color of fingernails is uniform and of a lighter tone than the skin on the back of the hand. The nail bed will show a pinkish color through the nail plate for the fair-skinned and a creamy beige for darker skin tones.

Discolored nails can give clues to internal body imbalances. If you notice an unexplained change in the color of your nails, it could be a sign of a health problem warranting a visit to your doctor. Toxicity to certain medications can also discolor nails.

♦ **Colorless** fingernails that appear much paler than the surrounding skin may indicate anemia.

♦ **Red or deep pink** fingernails can indicate a tendency to poor peripheral circulation.

♦ **Blue** nails may be a sign that the blood is not receiving adequate oxygen due to respiratory disorders, cardiovascular problems, or lupus erythematosus. Blue nails may also be a reaction to dyes or chemicals.

♦ **Yellow** nails may be the consequence of colored nail enamels, nail hardeners, tetracycline, fungus, diabetes, psoriasis, or heredity.

♦ **White, crumbly, soft** nails can result from a fungal infection leading to thickening and ridging of the fingernails. The fungus usually begins at the free edge of the nail and works its way down to the root.

♦ **Half white/half pink** nails may indicate a fungal infection or, more seriously, kidney disease.

♦ **Small white patches** that gradually move down the nail are usually a sign of injury to the nail matrix (such as bending the nail tip too far back) or of contact exposure to harsh soaps or cleaning products.

♦ **Purple or black** nails are usually due to trauma to the nail (hit the iron nail next time, not your keratin one!) or may also be a sign of vitamin B_{12} deficiency. However, a brown or black streak that begins at the base of the nail and extends to its tip could be a diagnostic clue to a potentially dangerous melanoma. See your healthcare provider to distinguish these streaks from a more serious medical problem.

SECRETS FOR NAIL FITNESS

◆ Try not to use your nails as tools. Fingernails are too special to be nature's screwdrivers.

◆ Always wear gloves while doing the dishes. Before putting on gloves, apply your favorite hand cream. The heat from the warm water will help your skin to absorb the cream. (This tip from Patricia Rivers-Sergienko.)

◆ To keep nails clean while doing dirty work, first scratch your nails over a bar of soap and then put on the appropriate gloves.

◆ It is much better to file your nails, but if you want to clip them, do so only when they are wet (after a shower or a bath).

◆ Clip baby's nails after a bath. Use blunt-end scissors and trim the nail in a curved edge following the natural shape. Press the tip of the finger down and out of the way as you cut.

◆ Gelatin and calcium supplements will not strengthen or harden your finger-nails. There is no substitute for eating fresh fruits, vegetables, and grains; drinking enough water every day; and getting basic exercise and proper rest.

CHAPTER 5
The Best Manicure

The activity of the hand runs through the whole history of man and the life history of the individual.
— Geza Revesz
The Human Hand: A Psychological Study

The history of manicuring nails can be traced back four thousand years to southern Babylon, where noblemen used solid gold implements to manicure their fingernails and toenails. It was common for military commanders in ancient Rome and Egypt to have their nails painted to match their lips before leaving for battle. In Egypt, highborn men and women used henna to stain their nails — the deeper the red, the more important the person. Today, nail polish for men is having a resurgence in popularity. It's being marketed as stylish, fun, and sexy. Colors are olive, khaki, and black. You may be skeptical now, but just think, there was doubt when earrings for men were reintroduced. And now they are dangling from many an ear.

FINGERNAIL POLISH

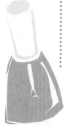

Coloring the nails goes back to the Ptolemaic period of ancient Egypt around 30 B.C.E., when the fingertips were dipped in orange henna.

It is believed that fingernail polish was invented by the Chinese about five thousand years ago. Royal Chinese colors for nails were red and black gloss. At that time, long nails were a sign that one had the means to be idle and therefore symbolized wealth. People took extreme care to protect each long nail; the fingertips were encased in a gold or silver sheath lined with soft material.

The History of
Nail Polish Ingredients

During the Ming Dynasty, nail polish was made of beeswax, egg whites, gelatin, vegetable dyes, and gum arabic collected from the bark of the wild acacia tree.

Jumping ahead to the twentieth century, here is an American recipe from 1910 for nail varnish. In this period of U.S. history, it was considered vulgar or tawdry to have painted nails. Tints were massaged into the fingernails, and varnish, applied with a camel's-hair brush, had a life span of only one day.

1910 NAIL VARNISH

This recipe comes from *Beauty Culture,* a 1910 publication by William A. Woodbury.

1 tablespoon (15 ml) tincture of benzoin (available at most pharmacies)
1 tablespoon (15 ml) 100-proof grain alcohol

To make and use:
"Mix and paint upon the nail with a fine camel-hair pencil, after the second polishing, allow to dry on. The resulting light gloss will remain on for at least a day."

THE BIRTH OF NAIL POLISH

You can thank Henry Ford and his automobiles for the development of nail polish. After World War I, there was a large supply of leftover nitrocellulose, which had been used for military explosives. By trial and error, a brave soul experimenting with the material discovered that boiling the nitrocellulose causes it to become soluble in organic solvents. When these solvents evaporate, the resulting material is a glossy, hard lacquer.

Around 1920, the automobile industry became interested in developing this unique lacquer process for painting new, assembly-line cars. Nitrocellulose lacquer was the paint of choice for Fords. Not long afterward, the beauty industry refined the lacquer formula by adding softening resins as the basis for nail polish.

Ingredients in Today's Nail Products

Today, the basic ingredient in nail lacquer is still nitrocellulose, in a solvent that evaporates easily. Most nail polishes are chemically identical. Plasticizers, resins, and color give the polish gloss, depth, and staying power. The manufacture of nail polishes requires attention to detail. The factory must be in a temperature-controlled, explosion-proof facility equipped with generators in case of power failure — the high vapor pressure of the substances used in nail polish and lacquers can lead to explosions.

Nail polishes make the existing nail plate harder but, to the best of our knowledge, do not affect the nail matrix, the source of new nails.

There are two ingredients — toluene and formaldehyde — found in most nail polishes today that can cause reactions in particularly sensitive individuals. If you think you needed to read labels only in the supermarket, think again. If you find yourself having a reaction to either of these two chemicals, you should abstain from using nail polishes that include these chemicals in their ingredients list.

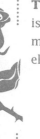

Toluene. Manufactured from petroleum by-products, toluene is one ingredient in nail polishes that can cause contact dermatitis. Many of the major cosmetic firms produce a nail enamel with a toluenesulfonamide, formaldehyde resin.

ALLERGY EVIDENCE

Allergic reactions to nail polish may surface first on your eyelids. If after applying a new nail polish your eyelids become red and swollen, this is your clue. Because eyelid skin is so delicate, it is particularly susceptible to contact dermatitis. (This means your nails or hands have rubbed your eyes.)

Formaldehyde. Commonly used in nail hardeners, formaldehyde is a chemical preservative that can cause skin irritation and allergic reactions. The first clue to a formaldehyde sensitivity may be a rash around the cuticles. However, dermatologists report that formaldehyde reactions can include anything from dry or discolored nails to bleeding under, or loss of, a nail.

Continuing to use products with formaldehyde after developing a sensitivity may lead to problems with the nails separating from the nail bed. If you are reactive to this preservative, look for polishes labeled "formaldehyde-free" or be careful that the polish does not touch the skin.

NATURAL HOME MANICURE

Taking care of your hard-working nails can be a relaxing, pleasant experience. Plan now to treat yourself to a scheduled home manicure every two weeks, and allow time for between-manicure touch-ups and nail maintenance as needed. (However, if a do-it-yourself manicure is not for you, you might still want to read through the following step-by-step instructions — they will help you decide the extent of a manicure you may want from a salon, as well as evaluate their techniques.) When done with a little care, a manicure will offer protection for your nails by eliminating rough edges, coating the nail surface, and helping to improve your self-image.

Manicures were first introduced in the United States in barbershops. The original barber chair was built with a hollow in each armrest with bowls for hand-soaking. During a routine haircut and shave, customers primed their nails for manicures.

Put on your favorite music. Cut some flowers from the garden or buy a bouquet. Take a lazy bath and set the mood for feeling good.

Before you begin your manicure, take a good look at your nails and hands. Now is the time to plan your strategy for maintaining healthy, strong, well-groomed nails. Are your nails dry? Do they have lines or ridges? Are the nails peeling in layers? Are they soft or brittle? In what shape are your cuticles? Are you a nail-biter and do you have hangnails? Have you been eating right and getting some exercise and enough sleep? If you don't take care of yourself, no one else will. Don't be overwhelmed. Learning to walk begins with the first step.

TOOLS FOR THE PERFECT HOME MANICURE

Good, focused work light

Hand towel: For drying your hands, and to place under your hand as you apply polish to your fingernails

100% cotton squares or balls: Useful for removing nail polish; cotton is very absorbent and does not leave behind bits of fiber

Polish remover without acetone: To remove any nail polish before manicure begins; try to find one without acetone, as it is damaging to the nail (see Step 1 to the right)

Finger bowl: For soaking fingernails

Warm water: To clean nails and soften cuticles so they can be gently pushed back, if necessary

Soft nail brush: To clean under and over your fingernails

New flexible nonmetal nail file: To lightly shape and smooth nail edges (should be new or sanitizable to prevent the spread of germs)

Natural nail oil or moisturizer: Nails have to be moisturized, just like skin

Orange stick: For gently pushing back the cuticle (was traditionally made of orange wood, although today you may find it made of flexible plastic)

Chamois-covered nail buffer (optional): Used to rub gently over bare nails, bringing out their natural shine

Nail powder (optional): To encourage a shine while buffing

Clear base coat: To provide a foundation for the nail polish

Clear or tinted nail polish: The main coat of polish (a clear polish will usually last longer without showing chips or peels)

Top coat: A protective, durable coating for the polish (may contain sunscreen)

Hand lotion: To promote supple skin by hydrating and moisturizing

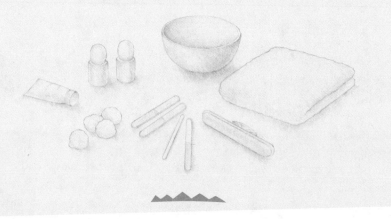

Step 1: Remove any polish from your nails

Partially saturate a cotton pad with the remover and work quickly to take up the old enamel. Start with the thumb. Use a cotton pad or swab to whisk off the polish with a rocking motion from the base of the nail to the tip. Do not smear the old polish into the cuticle or the surrounding tissues. Use this product sparingly and minimize skin contact. Never buy — and never be talked into using — a polish remover system that requires you to stick your entire finger into the jar of solution.

Polish removers are just not good for the nails. Avoid those containing acetone or chemical relatives of acetone, even if they say they have conditioners. This solvent degreases the nails, taking the oil out of them so that they cannot retain moisture. In addition, acetone and the alcohol in polish removers damage the surface of the nail, affect the nail's natural luster, and weaken and thin the nail plate. If you must use an acetone-based remover, dilute it with about 6 drops of olive or castor oil.

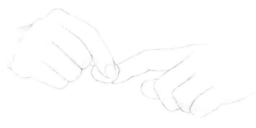

Step 2: Rinse

Rinse your fingernails in warm water immediately after using polish remover. Then scrub nails gently with a soft-bristle brush. Towel dry. If you apply moisturizer to your nails and hands while they are still a bit damp, it helps seal in the moisture.

If you've done this the night before the manicure, wear cotton gloves to bed for an extra skin treatment.

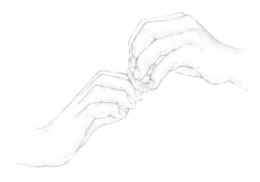

Step 3: File

Filing is necessary to shape and buff away any imperfections. File fingernails only when they are dry and free of cream.

When shaping nails, file from one edge of the nail to the center, and then from the other edge back to the center. Never file in the corners. Use long, smooth strokes and try not to saw the nail. Filing nails in the direction they grow prevents splitting.

For an easy filing position, make a fist and then uncurl your fingers slightly. File with your fingers facing you.

Keep your nails even and at a workable length for you. Softly square or oval tips are easier to maintain.

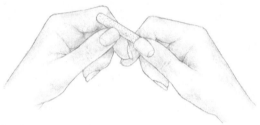

Step 4: Soak

Soak fingertips briefly in warm water after filing the nails. For a treat, try the Pineapple-Yogurt Nail Soak (see facing page), or, if you suffer from infected or irritated nails, see the recipe for the Warm Flower Soak on page 117.

Stained nails: If your nails are stained, now is a good time to soak them for 10 minutes in a solution of 1 capful of hydrogen peroxide to 1 cup (250 ml) of warm water. You can repeat this practice once a week. After the soak, use a soft nail brush and scrub under the free edge of each nail with baking soda and water.

TO AVOID PEELING NAILS

- To maintain shape and an even surface, file your nails with a fine-grit file or round nail disk.
- Never peel away a torn, chipped, or split nail. Instead, use scissors or a nail clipper and a fine-grit file. This is especially important for nail-biters.
- Don't allow your nails and cuticle area to become dry and rough. Try to apply a moisturizer or cuticle cream every time you wash your hands.

PINEAPPLE-YOGURT NAIL SOAK

This recipe is shared by Patricia Rivers-Sergienko, a natural nail care professional. Pineapple contains two helpful ingredients: bromelain, an enzyme that can reduce inflammation and pain, and alpha-hydroxy acids (AHAs), which peel off dead skin cells. Yogurt is very nourishing and a natural healer.

1/2 teaspoon (2.5 ml) apple cider vinegar

1 teaspoon (5 ml) olive oil

2 tablespoons (30 ml) pineapple juice, fresh or canned

2 tablespoons (30 ml) plain organic yogurt, regular or nonfat

To make:

1. Measure each ingredient and add to bowl.

2. Whip mixture with a fork until blended and creamy.

To use:

1. Dip fingers in the bowl and relax, allowing each hand to sit in the mixture for 5 minutes.

2. Massage both hands and fingers with the pineapple-yogurt mixture. Leave on skin for a few more minutes. Then rinse in warm water and pat dry. Use a fresh batch each time you do a manicure.

Step 5: Gently push back cuticles

Never cut your cuticles or push them back aggressively. The cuticle is the shield that protects the root of the nail — the matrix — from unfriendly bacteria and dirt. *Do not use cuticle removers.* Cuticle removers contain alkali and are among the harshest cosmetic products on a store's shelves. Regularly moisturizing the nail with an oil is a safer and more effective process for keeping the cuticles in good condition.

To gently push back the cuticle, use a soft, moist towel or an orange stick. Trim excess dead skin and hangnails with small, sharp scissors only when necessary. Never cut living skin.

Step 6: Clean under your nails

Avoid using a pointy or metal tool to clean under your nails. Instead, use a nail brush. Being too vigorous may create a space that allows fungi or bacteria to grow, so be gentle.

Step 7: Moisturize

Use a moisturizer on your cuticles, nails, and hands every time they have been in water. This is an ideal to work toward. The best store-bought skin moisturizer will contain phospholipids (natural emulsifiers and humectants), urea, and/or lactic acid. You can also try unrefined avocado oil or pure jojoba liquid. Or prepare a natural recipe such as Perfect Moisturizing Hand Cream (page 87).

Step 8: Massage

This is a good time to massage your hands. If you like, turn on some music that is soothing to your spirit. These strokes are adapted from those suggested by Michael Reed Gach, author of *Arthritis Relief at Your Fingertips*. Rub on a moisturizing cream, or mix 1 tablespoon (15 ml) of gently warmed avocado oil with 3 to 5 drops of your favorite pure essential oil and allow your hands to savor the experience.

Palm rub. Rub your palms together briskly to create some warmth, and then rub the backs of each hand.

Back of hands press. Clasp the fingers of both hands together with the palms facing. Squeeze the fingertips against the back of your hands. Hold for 5 to 10 seconds. Relax. Breathe deeply. Repeat.

web pinch

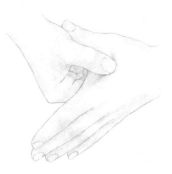

Web pinch. The space between each of your fingers is the web. Pinch between the thumb and the index finger, hold for a moment, then rub. Repeat this process between each of the fingers on both hands. Eastern therapies hold that applying pressure on the finger's web sites (not the Internet!) helps to dispel headaches and move toxins from the body.

Finger circles. Use your opposite hand to gently stretch and make little circles with each finger and thumb. Reverse direction of finger rotation. Repeat on the other hand.

Wrist compress. Support the wrist of one hand with the palm, fingers, and thumb of the other and squeeze lightly for about five seconds. Next, create the motion of a washing machine by gently rotating back and forth the wrist being held in the grasp of the supporting hand, while gently moving the holding hand in the opposite direction. Give the other wrist the same gentle treatment.

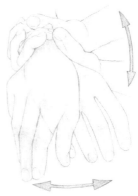

Forearm press. Knead the outer muscle of the forearm below the elbow. Push the tips of your four fingers sensitively into the skin, using the thumb as anchor, and work slowly up and down the arm, about three times, as if you were kneading bread dough. Repeat on the other arm.

wrist
compress

Elbow rub. Take this opportunity to moisturize the elbow and forearm with your favorite cream or lotion by massaging with the fingertips of the opposite hand in circular movements from the elbow down to the wrist, then over the hand and fingers.

Arm and finger stretch. Interlace the fingers of both hands with the palms facing and then slowly turn the palms outward. Stretch your arms in front of you and give the fingers and arms an easy, relaxed stretch. Release and shake out your hands as if you were trying to dry your nails.

Step 9: Apply polish

If you are going to use nail polish, wet a corner of a soft cotton towel and wipe any remaining cream from the nails. Pat dry.

The best way to apply nail polish is in three coats: a clear base coat followed by the polish, and topped with a clear top coat to lock in the color.

Applying nail polish can be tricky for the inexperienced, so here are some tips to start you off:

- ◆ Allow the clear base coat to dry for 3 minutes before applying the polish; this will act as a foundation for the polish and help to prevent nail stains caused by colored nail polish.
- ◆ Do the thumb last; it can be a helpful tool for mopping up polish spills on the cuticles of your other fingers.

- Blend nail polish by rolling the bottle between your palms. (Shaking causes air bubbles.)
- When you are applying polish, work in a well-ventilated room so that you will not breathe in the vapors.
- Using a clear polish rather than a colored one has its advantages — it shows less wear and doesn't have to be changed as often.
- Apply polish to the underside of the free edge of the nail, and then from the base of the nail to its free edge.
- Apply nail polish in two thin coats. Use three strokes from base to tip. First polish up the center, then up each side. Let the first layer dry for 3 minutes and the second for 5 minutes.
- Avoid quick-dry polishes; they most likely contain acetone, which can parch your nails. A thicker, slower-drying polish will hold the moisture and give your nails more flexibility.
- Brush on a top coat to lock in the color and protect the polish.

Note: Long-term use of colored polishes may discolor the natural nail.

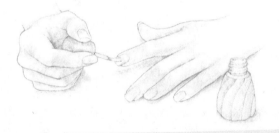

STAYING POWER

To increase the longevity of your nail polish application, before applying the first base coat, dip your unpolished fingernails into a mixture of white vinegar and warm water. Use this formula:

2 teaspoons (10 ml) white vinegar
1/2 cup (125 ml) warm water

Step 10: Buffing

If you decide you want an alternative to nail polish, try nail buffing. (It is not necessary to buff nails before applying polish.) Buffing will shine your nails, smooth away ridges, and improve circulation to the fingertips.

Use either a dry paste (see recipe for Tinted Nail Buffing Cream on page 112) or some light vegetable oil and a chamois-covered nail buffer.

For a natural gloss, buff the nails gently in one direction, with downward strokes from the base to the free edge of the nail. Raise the buffer after each stroke (otherwise you'll begin to feel a burning sensation). About 10 strokes lightly on each nail should be adequate.

Caution: Vigorous buffing, with heavy pressure, can cause ridges and thinning of the nails. If your nails are thin, limit buffing to once a month.

Caution for children: Do not buff children's nails — they have their own natural glow, and buffing can thin the nail's surface.

According to Beatrice Kaye, the original MGM movie studio manicurist, the rage in nail polish in 1924 was the "moon manicure." The free edge of the nail was point-shaped, and the polish was applied only to the center of the nail. The moon and the free edge of the fingernail were left uncovered.

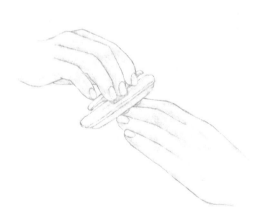

TINTED NAIL BUFFING CREAM

Alkanet, an important dye plant, is also known as dyer's or Spanish bugloss. It is a lovely perennial with a purple-brown root native to the eastern Mediterranean. The name comes from the Spanish *alcanna,* derived from an earlier Arabic word for henna.

½ cup (125 ml) sweet
   almond oil
1 tablespoon (15 ml)
   alkanet root, powdered
¼ ounce (7 g) beeswax
Up to 30 drops of essen-
   tial oils of your choice
   (for extravagant pam-
   pering, try a combina-
   tion of otto of rose
   and violet)

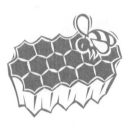

To make:

1. Pour the almond oil in a bottle or jar and add the powdered alkanet root. Stir together, and then seal, label, and refrigerate for two weeks. Gently shake the bottle daily.

2. After two weeks, the oil will be cranberry in color. Strain it through a coffee filter and bring to room temperature.

3. Melt the beeswax in a double boiler. Slowly stir in the alkanet oil. Remove from heat and add the essential oils of your choice.

4. Pour into cosmetic jars and label. Let sit overnight before using.

To use:

1. Spread a thin layer of the cream directly on the nails. Gently rub it in and leave undisturbed for a few minutes.

2. Buff with a nail buffer toward the free edge of the nail and lift the buffer after each stroke.

CHAPTER 6
Common Problems
and Everyday Remedies

▼▼▼▼▼

Only one thing can bring about
fresh change — new information!

— Anonymous

We rely on our fingernails for so many tasks that periodic maintenance is a must. This care can work to both prevent and relieve many common fingernail problems, such as nail- and cuticle-biting; bacterial, yeast, and fungal infections; and brittle or split nails. If done with care, this time spent may actually be enjoyable.

You can relieve or cure many fingernail problems with simple homemade natural remedies. However, for serious nail infections or lingering ailments, consult with a specialist first — it's a visit of value to prevent chronic, long-term fingernail problems.

NAIL- AND CUTICLE-BITING

"Don't bite the hand that feeds you." Nail-biters' nails are usually short and frayed, but the truth is that biting fingernails is thought to make them grow faster. This may often go unnoticed because nail-biters spend a great deal of time gnawing off fragments of past biting efforts.

Nail-biting and cuticle-biting sometimes go hand-in-hand. It's a difficult behavior to control but one worth changing, as it commonly causes deformed nails, raggedness, infection, hangnails, and warts. Stress — and how we deal with it — is often a factor in this habit. Sigmund Freud theorized that nail-biters are seeking satisfaction of some unfulfilled desire (probably the desire to have healthy, attractive nails and cuticles!). Whatever the reason, following are some tips on how to change this behavior and care for its destructive effects on fingernails.

NAIL-BITERS'
ALOE VERA OINTMENT

For as long as I can remember, I've heard tales of the old-fashioned reme-dy of coating the nails with a bad-tasting liquid polish. However, I have talked to numerous habitual nail-biters who have grown to love this bitter polish concoction.

A worthy alternative to the chemical polish product is a natural oint-ment made from the gel of fresh aloe vera leaves.

Several fresh leaves of the aloe vera plant

AMAZING ALOE

According to legend, aloe was one of the plants that grew in the Garden of Eden. This suc-culent, native to Africa, has a traditional use for healing wounds and as an antifungal agent. A multifunctional plant used for a wide range of basic first-aid purposes, its leaf produces a gel that is helpful for treating sunburn, wrinkles, insect bites, skin irritations, scarring, and minor cuts and scratches.

To cultivate aloe, plant in full sun. Water regularly, but allow the soil to dry out between waterings. In temperate cli-mates, you can grow aloe in a sunny window.

To make:
1. Cut a fresh aloe leaf down the center. With a spoon, scoop out the gel.
2. When you have collected a quantity of gel, place it in a double boiler. Boil the "sticky stuff" down to a thicker, pastelike consistency.
3. Spoon into a small clean jar with lid. Label, date, and store in a cool place.

To use:
When the urge arises to nibble on your fingernails, rub the aloe paste on the edges of the nails. The taste should discourage you.

Caution: A little bit of this gel goes a long way. Large internal doses of concen-trated aloe can cause vomiting. If you are pregnant and think you might be tempted to nibble despite the application of oint-ment, avoid this remedy, as the plant's anthraquinone glycosides are purgative.

For infected nails: Try a warm com-press of fresh aloe vera gel. Squeeze the gel directly on the infected finger and cover with a warm, slightly damp cotton cloth.

Caring for Your Hangnails

Hangnails, fleshy bits of dry skin that have split away from the edges of the fingernail, are very common in nail-biters. They can be painful and become a site for secondary infections. Children often have hangnails. This is a good time to give them some direction on how to keep their skin and nails fit. Suggest that they resist the temptation to tear off a hangnail. If it's in the way, cut the flap of skin at its base with clippers or small scissors. Store a bottle or tube of hand cream at every sink and try to get the family in the habit of using it after hand washing. Hangnails can also signal dry cuticles caused by frequent hand washing, cold weather, or rough working conditions. Moisturize the nails and skin around them often. Regularly moisturizing the cuticle area will help cut down on the urge to bite.

Nail Tips, or Caps, for Nail-Biters

In the old days, the remedy for biting nails was a piece of red flannel tied around the most bitten fingers. Today, a more cosmetically appealing alternative is nail tips, or caps, applied to thicken the nail edges. Nail tips are synthetic white nail edges that are tailored to have a natural nail width and arch. They are applied with a coat of adhesive to the free edge of the fingernail. This change in density at the nail point seems to alert nail-biters to reconsider their actions.

If the aloe ointment isn't working, you might want to try a nail-tips remedy for three months. It may be just enough to change the nail-biting habit and relieve the possibility of continual infections around the nails.

Caution: Never apply an artificial nail if the tissue around the natural nail is infected or irritated. Wait until this area is completely healed. Then permit a month's rest for your nails after each three-month period with synthetic nails.

MORE TIME-TESTED IDEAS TO CURB NAIL-BITING

- Sit on your hands when you have the urge to bite your fingernails.
- Clench your fists for a minute.
- Put moisture back — apply cuticle and nail cream as often as you wash your hands.
- Carry a low-grit nail file to smooth rough edges.
- Wear gloves.
- Try acupuncture, hypnotism, or behavioral therapy.

Regular Manicures

Regular home or salon manicures can also help you to break the nail-biting habit. Having attractive hands may act as an incentive to use those "pearly whites" (teeth, that is) for something other than shaping fingernails. (See chapter 5, "The Best Manicure," beginning on page 100.)

NAIL INFECTIONS

Chronic infection of the skin around a fingernail can be due to many causes and is always an uncomfortable condition. A new medical term you may hear is *paronychia,* but the problem has probably bothered folks since caveperson days. An older name for this condition is *whitlow.* Whatever the name, the definition is the same: a break in the skin resulting in a painful inflammation and infection of a finger or toe, directly behind the cuticle or around the nail fold. The area is usually tender, swollen, red, and infected. Pus may be noticeable.

Paronychia can be caused by a bacterial (*Staphylococcus aureus* or *Streptococcus*) or yeast *(Candida)* infection that attacks growing tissue at the base of the nails. The nail plate may show white, rippled, horizontal lines, called Beau's lines, which mark a temporary disturbance in the nail's growth. Thumb-suckers, nail-biters, and nail- or cuticle-pickers are prone to this condition.

If you have an infected nail, visit a dermatologist to have the type of infection analyzed (yeast vs. bacterial), as this will help you get the appropriate treatment. Depending on the cause, remedies could include antibacterial or antifungal agents.

Vitamin Therapy

At the first sign of a nail or skin infection, reach for some helpful vitamins to take daily with meals until the problem has been resolved. I take B-complex vitamins, essential for natural cortisone production — folic acid, niacin, biotin, and 100 to 300 mg pantothenic acid — one-third dose with each meal, plus vitamin C (up to 1000 mg a day). Vitamin C stimulates the production of antibodies and speeds the healing process.

Herbal Remedies

There are also several soothing herbal preparations you can use to treat fingernail infections. As with all ailments, if the problem seems especially serious or is persistent, check in with a specialist or physician for treatment or advice.

WARM FLOWER SOAK

This infusion of lavender or chamomile will help soothe and reduce skin irritations and inflammation. Lavender also helps inhibit bacteria.

1 quart (1 liter) clear soft water or distilled water

2 ounces (56 g) dried German chamomile or lavender flowers

1 teaspoon (5 ml) essential oils of rosemary, lavender, grapefruit, or geranium (optional)

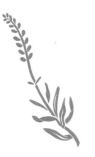

To make:
1. Boil the water and pour, still steaming, over the dried herbs.
2. Steep the flowers in a covered pot (about 20–30 minutes).
3. When the water has cooled to a comfortable temperature, strain the flowers and pour some of the liquid into a small bowl. Or, if you like, save the blossoms and let your fingers play with them while they are immersed in this infusion. If desired, add the essential oils, using any single oil or combination.

To use:
Soak the infected finger for at least 10 minutes, two or three times a day. If you like, re-warm to a comfortable temperature each time you do a soak.
Note: Save the remaining, unused liquid in a closed container in the refrigerator for the next dip; it will keep for about two weeks.
Caution: Those with ragweed allergies may be sensitive to chamomile blossoms.

ANTISEPTIC SOAK

For nail infections that are not healing readily, this regimen may be an alternative approach until you can see your healthcare provider.

2 quarts (2 liters) soft water

1 tablespoon (15 ml) bleach

A few drops mild liquid soap

To make:
1. Boil the water and add the bleach and the liquid soap.
2. Stir with a wooden spoon.
3. Pour 1 cup of this mixture into a small glass bowl and cool to a comfortable temperature.
4. Bottle and label the remaining liquid.

To use:
1. Soak the infected finger three times a day for 10 minutes. You might want to gently warm the bottled liquid in a warm-water bath each time.
2. Repeat this procedure for four days (or longer if the wound has not healed).

PROTECTING NAIL INFECTIONS

When you have an infection around your nails, wear protective gloves to do wet work on such tasks as washing dishes, cars, laundry, and gardening. Turn the gloves inside out and wash them at least once a week. When the infection is gone, toss the gloves. (It's akin to changing your toothbrush after the flu.) For more about gloves, see "If the Glove Fits, Wear It," on page 80.

VERBENA COMPRESS

From the twelfth century, here is Saint Hildegard of Bingen's Verbena Remedy for soothing a whitlow (an infected nail).

Vervain, also known as verbena, has been associated with magic since the time of the Druids. Pliny, A.D. 77, wrote that "people who have been rubbed with it will obtain their wishes, banish fever . . . and cure all disease." With that kind of endorsement, this herb belongs in everyone's garden. Verbena is an astringent and aids in the healing of open wounds.

1 tablespoon (15 ml)
verbena leaves and
flowers, dried and
ground
Spring water to cover

To make:

1. With mortar and pestle, pound the dried verbena to break out its essence.

2. Place the crushed verbena in a small muslin sack with a drawstring. Drop into boiling water and boil for 3 minutes.

3. Press the excess water from the sack and place the muslin with the warm herb on a small, clean, ironed piece of linen large enough to cover the infected finger.

To use:

Wrap the cloth with the herb-filled sack around the finger and leave this compress on until the sack loses its heat. Repeat as needed.

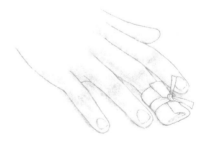

LEMON FOLK REMEDY

In addition to relieving the pain of infection, this treatment will remove stains from your nails. A bonus is that lemon juice restores the natural pH of your skin.

1 or 2 fresh lemons

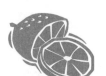

To use:
1. Cut a small opening at the end of a lemon and push in the affected finger.
2. Keep the infected finger in place until the lemon ceases to draw (stops stinging). If you wish, apply another lemon until the pain is relieved.
Note: If the infection or inflammation continues for a time, the nail will lose luster and have ridges, and the developing nail will be affected. When home remedies don't work, it's time to consult a dermatologist who specializes in nail problems.

SKIN AND PH

The abbreviation pH stands for "potential hydrogen," but it is commonly used to measure the alkalinity or acidity of a substance. A pH of 7.0 is the neutral point; the neutral range is considered to be 6.5 to 7.5. Water and blood are usually in the neutral range. Above 7.0 alkalinity increases; below 7.0 acidity increases. Lemon juice and vinegar are mildly acidic, with a pH between 2.0 and 3.0. The pH of the hair and skin is around 5.0, slightly acidic.

Most good, natural skin cleansers, hair conditioners, and moisturizers have a pH between 3.5 and 5.5, so as not to irritate the skin. Natural ingredients, with their own natural pH, make the best cosmetics for your skin.

BRITTLE, SPLIT NAILS

The medical term for this problem (yes, there is a medical term) is *onychorrhexis,* splitting and brittleness of the nails. The exact causes of this condition are not known. When hands are frequently in hot water and in contact with harsh soaps, detergents, or other irritating substances, nails take the punishment. Frequent use of polish remover, which dries out the nail bed, is another common culprit.

Here's the explanation. When hands are immersed in water, the nail cells swell. Then when the nails dry, the cells shrink. With repeated swelling and shrinking, the nail will eventually split. Contrary to current opinion, the problem is not due to lack of protein, gelatin, calcium, or vitamins. There is not much calcium in the nail; its hardness is due to its special protein bonds. Extra protein or gelatin in the diet will not make our nails harder.

The best way to prevent fingernails from splitting is to keep your hands away from hot water, drying soaps, and detergents. Apply nail oil or cream often. Wear waterproof gloves for wet tasks. Cotton-lined gloves or a separate pair of cotton gloves inside rubber or vinyl gloves may offer the most protection. There are hypoallergenic gloves available now for those sensitive to latex, made from a material called nitrile™ that resists bleach and household solvents. If these methods fail, what follows are some easy remedies to help brittle nails.

Salad hands. Mediterranean chefs use this remedy every time they make a salad. They rub the olive or avocado oil from the dressing into their nails and cuticles. Massaging the cuticle area increases circulation and encourages new nail growth. The oil seals in the moisture that is depleted when hands are in and out of water.

Did you know that because the nail is so porous, it gives off moisture a hundred times as fast as the skin?

Thuja. A homeopathic remedy for brittle nails is Thuja 6x. You should be able to obtain this treatment in stores selling medicinal herbs or from a homeopathic specialist.

Thuja 6x is made from the fresh, green twigs of the American arborvitae or Eastern white cedar. These branches contain thujone, a volatile oil that is said to affect the concentration of salt, water, and electrolytes in the body, as well as other wax, resin, and gelatinous ingredients. It encourages moisturization and helps prevent and heal brittle or split nails. Thuja is best in a homeopathic, diluted dose because it can be toxic when taken at full strength and in excess.

Caution: Pregnant women and people with irritant, dry coughs should not take thuja.

WHAT IS HOMEOPATHY?

The practice of homeopathy is centered on the belief *similia similibus curentur,* meaning "like cures like." Homeopathic practitioners use herbs, minerals, and animal extracts for their medicines. Homeopathic treatments involve the administration of minute diluted doses. For instance, if you were bitten by a snake, a homeopathic remedy might be a very dilute extract of snake venom.

A homeopathic remedy is first prepared in a solution as the "mother tincture." A small quantity is then diluted to one tenth (by the addition of nine parts alcohol or water) and shaken vigorously. A small quantity of this preparation is then diluted again to one tenth and shaken. This process is repeated again and again, producing weaker and weaker solutions identified as 3X (diluted three times), 6X (diluted six times), 30X (diluted thirty times), and so on, according to the number of dilutions.

HENNA NAIL PASTE

Henna has wonderful conditioning and nail-strengthening properties. This is a fun, natural nail treatment to do with children or on your own.

½ cup (125 ml) boiled water

½ teaspoon (2.5 ml) uncolored, neutral henna powder

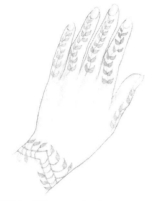

Mehndi henna design

To make:

1. Add the henna to the warm, boiled water and mix well, using a non-metal stirring spoon.

2. Make a paste of the mixture and place it in a small jar with a screw-top lid.

To use:

1. Using a chopstick, glob the henna paste on each of your clean, dry nails. Even though the henna is neutral, the color will be a soft green. This green will not remain on your nails, and it will not stain.

2. Let the henna paste dry on your nails and cuticles for 10 minutes. You will feel a pleasant "drawing" sensation.

3. Afterward, rinse your fingers, towel dry, and gently buff the nails.

4. You can use neutral henna once or twice a week for nail conditioning. Remember to stir the henna mixture each time.

MEHNDI: BODY ART WITH HENNA

Mehndi is the 5000-year-old traditional art of adorning the fingers, hands, forearms, toes, and shins with a non-permanent dye paste made from the leaves of the henna plant. Hand and body henna designs vary from large floral patterns in Arab countries to fine, lacy paisleys in India to bold geometric patterns in Africa. Henna designs will usually last for 4 to 6 weeks.

Painting with henna is more than a decorative art. In some countries people believe it to have healing properties, and it is used in place of gloves; in others, there is a mystical, protective connotation allied with its use, especially in marriage rituals.

SOOTHING NAIL AND CUTICLE OIL

Treat yourself to a warm, relaxing nail oil bath at least twice a week. Almond oil is a good base moisturizer for brittle or split nails. You can add the essential oils of sage, chamomile, lavender, or vanilla-like benzoin as helpful agents against any fungal infections or bacteria that might be hiding around the cuticles and under the nails. These oils also add a bit of aromatherapy to enhance your mood.

4 tablespoons
(60 ml) pure
sweet almond oil
20–25 drops of your
choice of essential oil
of sage, chamomile,
lavender, or benzoin
1 vitamin E capsule
(400 IU)

To make:

1. Pour the almond oil into a small bottle and add the essential oil of your choice.

2. Pierce a vitamin E capsule and squeeze it into the mixture. Shake thoroughly.

3. Label the bottle with the contents and the date you created the blend.

To use:

1. When you are ready to use the blended oil, warm the bottle by setting it in a bowl of hot water for a few minutes.

2. Soak your nails in the blended oil for 10 minutes.

3. Sleep with cotton gloves on or wrap the hands in plastic wrap covered with a towel for at least 30 minutes for extra benefit.

For a massage: Give yourself or someone you look after a nail and hand massage before bedtime. Rub a few drops of the oil into the nails, cuticles, and skin. At the end of the massage, have the recipient rub his/her hands together, breathe deeply, and rest. The massage is relaxing and at the same time will stimulate circulation in the hands.

Caution: Essential oil of lavender is not recommended for those in the first trimester of pregnancy or who have very low blood pressure.

ALMOND JOY

Eat 6 raw almonds every day to relieve splitting of the fingernails. Linoleic acid, an essential fatty acid (EFA), is one of the important components of almonds. Among other benefits, EFAs help lubricate the body's cells.

HORSETAIL NAIL BATH

With a high content of silicic acid (5 to 8 percent), horsetail is a good astringent, antiseptic, and tissue and nail strengthener. On the days you are not using cuticle and nail oils, bathe your fingernails in this decoction of horsetail. Try this regimen over several months: one week of nail oil treatments alternating with one week of horsetail nail baths.

1 ounce (28 g) fresh horsetail in 1-inch (2.5 cm) pieces, sliced and bruised (or use the dried herb, cut and sifted)

Cold spring water to cover, about 1 pint (½ liter)

3 teaspoons (15 ml) sugar (helps extract the silicon from the herb)

To make:

1. In a small pot with lid, cover the horsetail with water, add the sugar, and simmer for 30 minutes.

2. Let the decoction cool to a comfortable temperature.

To use:

Soak fingernails for 10 minutes.

HORSETAIL TEA FOR BRITTLE NAILS

When you want to attack the problem from both the inside and the outside, drink horsetail tea and use the Horsetail Nail Bath (above).

This is the way Jim Duke, author of *The Green Pharmacy,* prepares the brew.

2 teaspoons (10 ml) dried stems of horsetail herb

2 cups (500 ml) water

2 teaspoons (10 ml) sugar (helps extract the silicon from the herb)

To make:

1. Put the horsetail in a stainless pot.

2. Cover with water and add the sugar. Bring to a boil and simmer for 3 hours.

3. Strain the liquid.

To use:

Drink 2 cups of the tea a day. You can double the amount of the recipe and store in the refrigerator; however, herbal water infusions and decoctions are best when fresh and should be used within one week.

BURDOCK SEED NAIL AND CUTICLE CONDITIONER

This recipe for an infused burdock seed oil is shared by Matthias Reisen of Healing Spirits Herb Farm in Avoca, New York. If you like going for extended walks and want to try your hand at wildcrafting (finding your own naturally grown herbs), start at the top. If you use purchased burdock seeds, skip ahead to the "To make:" section on the next page.

Burdock's effects on the skin have been valued from China to Chile, from Canada to Russia. The plant contains inulin, an essential oil, B-vitamins, and fatty acids. The seeds have a demulcent nature and help to restore smoothness to the skin and nails. Burdock is also an alterative and is suggested for treating chronic skin diseases.

Burdock seeds
Cold-pressed olive oil
Liquid contents of a 400 IU
   vitamin E capsule
   (optional)

To keep nails and cuticles in top form, some fashion models save empty, clean nail polish bottles and fill them with a light vegetable oil. They then brush this oil on their nails and cuticles several times during the day.

Wildcrafting and harvesting burdock:
If you've decided to collect your own *Arctium lappa* burrs, wear heavy-duty rubber gloves — these guys are clingers! Take a field guide to properly identify the plant.
1. Run your gloved hand up the stock and remove only the marble-size burrs. Put the burrs in a heavy-weight paper shopping bag or a woven plastic feed sack.
2. Wearing thick-soled shoes or boots, place the bag on a concrete floor or other hard surface. "Stomp" or crush the plant material, stepping heavily or jumping (you can also use a large mallet). This process is fun when you want to get rid of your aggressions (and have plenty of time). The seeds will come loose.
3. Shake the contents of the bag onto a metal ⅛" mesh screen, resting on a bucket filled with cold water.
4. Sift the tiny seeds into the bucket. The seeds will fall to the bottom. Discard the floating material and strain the water with a fine sieve to catch the seeds.
5. Place the wet seeds on a screen to dry for about 48 hours.

To make:

1. Grind the seeds once they are dry. (You may have the most success using a Japanese ceramic mortar, or *saribachi,* with a wooden pestle, or *suri kogi,* or using a stone mortar and pestle — see Resources.

2. Put the ground seeds into a mason jar. Fill the jar with enough olive oil to cover the seeds with about an inch to spare.

3. Lightly screw on the lid (not tight) or cover the jar with a double fold of cheesecloth secured with a rubber band. Label the jar with contents and date, and then place the covered jar in a paper bag and set in a sunny window for two weeks.

4. Strain well twice, using a metal strainer lined with cheese-cloth or an unbleached paper coffee filter, to remove all bits of plant material.

5. Simply decant (pour off) the oil into dark-colored bottles, taking care not to allow any sediment to enter your new bottles.

6. If you wish, add a few drops of vitamin E oil as a preservative.

7. Cork or screw on a lid. Label the new bottles with the name of the herb and the date the oil was prepared.

To use:

Rub the oil into your cuticles and fingernails. Burdock seed oil is also good for dry scaly skin, cradle cap, eczema, and psoriasis.

WILDCRAFTING TIPS

♦ Be familiar with, or bring someone who is familiar with, the terrain. Do not harvest plants that may have been sprayed with toxic pesticides.

♦ Do not harvest plants that are near busy highways.

♦ Bring field guides to help you identify plants. Sometimes the variations within plant species are subtle. Part of the fun of learning about herbs and plants is becoming aware of the amazing adaptations that have occurred to ensure the plant's survival.

♦ Do not overharvest plant populations; pick sparingly, and leave plenty of each species in its natural habitat to sustain its population.

♦ Be aware of what plants and herbs are endangered and are struggling for survival in the wild; in these cases, you may wish not to wildcraft but to purchase the plant or herb, and to verify with the supplier that the plant was obtained in a responsible manner.

NAIL POLISH TIPS FOR NAILS THAT SPLIT

◆ A coating of clear nail polish, or a formalin-free nail hardener, helps to keep the fingernail from splitting further. For greater durability, also apply a thin line of polish on the underneath of the free edge of the nail.

◆ Nail polish removers dry the nail and are really the bad guys of manicures. To cut down on the use of polish removers, make a practice of applying a new coat of polish over the old coat at least once before starting fresh.

◆ Use colored nail polishes only for special occasions to cut down on the chipped-nails, must-remove-polish syndrome.

NAIL FUNGUS

How does a fungus produce an infection? Nail fungi invade the superficial layers of the skin and in a few days germinate their spores along the edge of fingernails or toenails. A mass of fungal filaments grows into the nails. Fungi love to eat protein or keratin. Our nails become the "fertilizer" for these skin fungi, and our sweat glands provide the moisture to irrigate the crop.

Not everyone who comes in contact with fungi becomes infected. General health and nutrition play a role, as well as good hygiene practices. Scratching fungal infections on other places on your body such as your scalp or beard, or ringworm on your chest, or scratching pets with a skin condition can spread the problem to your fingernails.

The first step in treating a nail fungal infection is to have it diagnosed correctly. Once you know what you're dealing with, you can take the appropriate steps to treat it.

Tinea Fungal Infections

Fungal infections of the nails (*Tinea unguium*) will begin at the ends of the nails and then spread to occupy the entire nail bed. Over time the nail degenerates, becoming thickened, crumbly, white, or yellow. It can be painful, but is most often only unsightly. Those who tend to pick up athlete's foot may also be prone to develop *Tinea* infections on their fingernails. (Why is it that when we read about or write about things like this, we develop an incredible urge to scratch?)

To fight a *Tinea* fungal infection of the nail:

◆ First, have it diagnosed correctly.
◆ Add fresh garlic to your diet (5 cloves a day).
◆ Take tincture of echinacea daily; this herbal remedy helps the body rid itself of microbial infections.
◆ Keep your nails short and dry.
◆ Wear gloves for wet tasks.
◆ Clean under and around your nails with non-distilled witch hazel extract.
◆ Apply the Nail-Biters' Aloe Vera Ointment on the affected area (see page 114).
◆ Try several herbal, antifungal remedies individually until you find the one that works for you (see page 130).

Candida nail infections

Candida are a specific genus of yeastlike fungi. A *Candida* nail infection may look like a *Tinea* infection, but it may also have a creamy discharge. This kind of infection seems to attack those who frequently have their hands in soapy water without gloves. Generally, these nail infections are slow in healing but will respond to some form of antifungal cream or treatment.

The yeast species in food has nothing to do with the *Candida* that infect the skin. Changing to a yeast-free diet will not help cure a *Candida* infection of the nails.

To fight a *Candida* infection of the nail:

◆ Keep your nails short.
◆ Take B vitamins. Add wheat germ and yogurt with active cultures to your diet.
◆ Keep your hands out of water (what a great excuse to get the family to help out here!) or wear protective gloves.
◆ Use your hair dryer to blow warm air under the edge of the nails a couple of times a day to keep them dry.

Herbal Antifungal Remedies

Following are three herbal antifungal remedies in three types of delivery systems: a wash or soak, an essential oil, and a glycerin tincture. If you have a stubborn fungal infection of your fingernails, try each one of these recipes individually to see which works best for you. Tea tree oil may be the easiest to find, so start there. Improvement happens slowly with fungal infections; even prescription medications can take six months to a year to work.

RED CEDAR GLYCERIN TINCTURE

The red cedar, named for its cinnamon red bark that becomes gray-brown over time, is native to northwest America. Red cedar leaves have strong antifungal, antibacterial, and immunostimulant properties.

1 part red cedar leaves, crushed

2 parts glycerin mixture (50% glycerin, 40% water, 10% ethyl alcohol or vodka)

To make:

1. Put the crushed red cedar leaves in a jar and cover with the appropriate amounts of glycerin, water, and alcohol.

2. Seal the jar, label, and store in a cool place for two weeks. Give the jar a turn every day, if possible.

3. After two weeks, strain twice through cheesecloth, pressing the liquid from the leaves.

4. Pour the strained liquid into clean, dark glass bottles. Seal and label.

To use:

Apply the tincture two to three times a day, with consistency, on the cuticle and under the free edge of the nail. You should begin to see some improvement at the end of one week.

Caution: Red cedar is not suggested for use during pregnancy or by those with kidney weakness.

MYRRH WASH OR SOAK

Myrrh, a bushy shrub native to Somalia and Saudi Arabia, has been prized for centuries for its fragrance and usefulness in cleansing and healing wounds. It is also considered an immune stimulant and an antifungal. You may even notice myrrh today as an astringent ingredient in mouthwashes and gargles for sore throat and mouth ulcers.

10 drops essential oil of myrrh or 2 teaspoons (10 ml) tincture of myrrh (see recipe below)

5 tablespoons (75 ml) comfortably warm spring water

To make:
Add the essential oil or tincture of myrrh to the warm water and stir well.

To use:
Use as a soak or a wash around and under the nails.

For stubborn infections: Take a tincture of myrrh (see recipe below) internally, 20 drops (1 ml) well diluted in half a glass of liquid, such as apple juice, three times a day with meals. (Myrrh is not noted for its pleasant taste.) Or take one 200 mg capsule three times a day.

Caution: If you are pregnant, avoid the use of myrrh, as it is also considered a uterine stimulant.

TINCTURE OF MYRRH

It is easy and inexpensive to make your own myrrh extract.

¼ cup (60 ml) crushed myrrh resin (available at most herb shops or wherever bulk herbs are sold)

¼ cup (60 ml) distilled water

¼ cup (60 ml) 190-proof grain alcohol

To make:
1. Combine the ingredients in a clean 6–8 ounce jar with a screw-top lid. Seal and label.
2. Steep for 3 to 4 weeks in a cool, dark place, turning daily.
3. Strain and rebottle in dark glass containers.

TEA TREE OIL DIRECT

The oil of tea tree is a broad-spectrum fungicide as well as an antibacterial and antiviral agent. It is also a soothing topical anesthetic. The clear, light, lemon-colored oil is best when packaged in amber or opaque containers to prevent chemical breakdown by light.

Essential oil of tea tree
Cotton swabs

To use:

1. For fungal infections of the nail, paint tea tree essential oil on clean, dry nails.

2. Use a cotton swab to dab the oil directly on the cuticle and under the free edge of the nail three times daily. Or massage the oil into the nail bed twice daily.

Caution: Some people are sensitive to tea tree oil. Try a patch test first on a small spot of non-infected skin. If your skin is reactive to full-strength tea tree oil, wash the area with soap and water. Then try cutting the strength of the essential oil by putting about 2 tablespoons of almond oil in a small glass bottle with 10 drops of tea tree oil. Shake well and paint around nails. Do not use tea tree oil near your eyes.

THE VERSATILE TEA TREE

The Australian aboriginal people have made use of the Melaleuca tree for at least a thousand years. They prepare a tea from the leaves, and make a leaf poultice remedy to apply directly to wounds. Following their example, during World War II Australian troops carried essential oil of tea tree in their first-aid kits as a powerful antiseptic, fungicide, and analgesic for cuts, abrasions, minor burns, toothaches, warts, and cold sores. Thursday Plantation was the first Australian company to commercialize the planting and growing of Melaleuca trees in New South Wales.

COOL POTATO BURN RELIEF

A burn pulls moisture from the skin. Applying fresh slices of potato to the burn is very cooling, and the skin will "drink" in the moisture. In addition, when I have used this remedy, I've had very little scarring after the burn had healed.

1 raw potato

To make:
Peel a raw potato and cut it into thin slices, or pulp it with a hand grater or food processor.

To use:
1. Apply the potato slices or raw pulp to soothe minor burns, an itchy rash, or bruises.
2. Apply fresh slices or pulp as each becomes dry.

LAVENDER FLOWER WASH

This infusion of lavender will help soothe and reduce redness and inflammation. Lavender also helps inhibit bacteria.

¼ cup (60 ml) fresh or dried lavender flowers
2 cups (500 ml) distilled water
½ tablespoon (7.5 ml) tincture of benzoin (available at most pharmacies) or 10 drops essential oil of lavender (optional)

To make:
1. Bruise the flowers with the back of a flat wooden paddle.
2. Simmer the flowers gently in distilled water (to cover) for 20 minutes or place in a covered jar with distilled water in a sunny window for an afternoon.
3. Strain through cheesecloth and store in a closed glass bottle in the refrigerator.
4. If you do not plan to use the flower water within a few days, add tincture of benzoin or 10 drops of essential oil of lavender. Shake well.

To use:
Pat on burn and repeat as necessary.

CHAPPED, CRACKED, RED, ROUGH HANDS

What it is: There are various opinions about the causes of chapped skin. The most logical explanation is overexposure of the hands to cold weather or low dew points (humidity). Another cause of chapping is repeated washing of the hands with harsh detergents. This not only chaps the hands but also allows fissuring so that contact irritants can gain entrance to the skin. Dry, chapped skin can also be one of the first signs of a vitamin A deficiency.

Suggested remedies: The most obvious remedy for chapped, cracked hands is moisturizer — and lots of it! There are several recipes listed below. However, you also want to find out why your hands are becoming so dry and chapped. If constant washing or overexposure is necessary given your job or living circumstances, moisturizer may be your only hope (although you should certainly wear gloves whenever possible). However, it may be that you suffer from a vitamin deficiency or you haven't been caring for your hands, in which case you should take preventive measures to guard against painfully cracked hands.

Vitamin therapy. One of the first signs of a vitamin A deficiency may be continually dry or chapped hands. Are carrots, sweet potatoes, and tomatoes on the menu? Do you have sandpaper skin or "gooseflesh" on the outer aspect of your arms and legs that does not go away? If you have these bumps on the outside of your thighs, check with your healthcare practitioner about the possibility of taking daily vitamin A supplements.

If you have been on a stringent diet and eliminated most fats from your menu, you may also be lacking in vitamin E. Add 2 tablespoons (30 ml) daily of wheat germ or an unsaturated oil like corn oil — both of which are rich in vitamin E — to your diet. Once your skin returns to its soft, lovable self, you can gradually reduce the amount of oil or wheat germ.

SPECIAL WASH FOR CHAPPED HANDS

This is a gentle cleanser that should not be irritating to the skin. If you repeat this regimen day and night several times a week, your chapped hands will become a thing of the past.

(The cornmeal accomplishes by a gentle abrasive action what a harsh soap does by chemical action. The cornmeal, however, does not draw all the moisture away from the important lower layers of the skin.)

1 small cucumber
½ tablespoon (7.5 ml) honey
Warm water
Mild soap — fine castile or Dove or Neutrogena
1 tablespoon (15 ml) cornmeal

To make:

1. Peel the cucumber and remove the seeds; blend or juice the vegetable for a few seconds. Mix with the honey and set aside in a small bowl.

2. Make a cornmeal paste by mixing warm water, soap, and cornmeal.

To use:

1. Wash your hands thoroughly with the cornmeal paste. Then rinse hands well in clean, warm (not hot) water. This helps to remove flaking skin cells and any soluble environmental pollutants.

2. While your hands are damp, apply the cucumber juice and honey mixture. Have someone help you wrap your hands in plastic wrap or insert them in large, zip-seal plastic bags. Cover with a towel, then relax as long as possible.

3. Rinse and dry hands. Apply moisture cream. If you've done this at night, wear loose-fitting cotton gloves to bed. (Wash the gloves regularly.)

4. Repeat cornmeal wash daily (and repeat as often as you can for badly chapped hands). In cold weather, substitute a *cold* water rinse in the morning to acclimate hands to cooler conditions. Dry well, then rub in a moisturizing cream.

ALMONDS, COMFREY, AND HONEY SOOTHING OINTMENT

Here is a recipe from the Middle Ages for painfully cracked hands. Almonds are known for their mildness and softening action on the skin. Comfrey, also known as bruisewort or knitbone, has been cultivated in gardens for centuries for the wound-healing qualities of the root and leaves. Allantoin, one of the constituents of comfrey, encourages healthy skin regrowth by stimulating cells, and also relieves itching.

1 ounce (28 g) ground almonds
1 egg, beaten
1/4 ounce (7 g) ground comfrey root
1 tablespoon (15 ml) honey

To make:
Combine well the almonds, egg, comfrey root, and honey, stirring with your hands or a wooden spoon. Refrigerate. (Of course, they didn't have refrigerators in the Middle Ages.)

To use:
1. Before bed, smooth this mixture over your hands and fingers and pull on either a pair of cotton gloves or old leather gloves. Follow this regimen for seven nights.

2. Each morning, rinse your hands and the gloves and apply a skin lotion. After the nightly routine of the first week, cut back to a once-a-week schedule for a month, and then repeat this recipe only on a monthly basis.

Caution: Internal use of comfrey is not recommended.

RED HANDS TIP

You can whiten red hands by rubbing them several times a day with a mixture of egg white and glycerin. At night, wear gloves to bed.

"SPRAINS A DRAIN" COMPRESS

This is a soothing herbal remedy that is very effective on a sprain. Both St.-John's-wort oil and arnica extract are worth having in your home or travel first-aid kit. First apply ice to the sprained finger, wrist, or elbow to minimize swelling, and then wrap in this compress.

1–4 teaspoons (5–20 ml) arnica extract

2 cups (500 ml) hot water

Burdock leaves or green cabbage leaves

2 cups (500 ml) boiling water

St.-John's-wort oil

To make:

1. Prepare a solution of arnica and hot water. A standard infusion is 1 to 4 teaspoons (5 to 20 ml) extract in 2 cups (500 ml) hot water.

2. Pound the fresh burdock or cabbage leaves, and then immerse them in boiling water for 2 minutes. Drain leaves on paper towels.

To use:

1. Coat the skin of the sprained area with St.-John's-wort oil.

2. Dip a soft, thin towel in the warm arnica wash. Squeeze out excess liquid and apply the towel to the sprain.

3. Cover with the warm wilted burdock or green cabbage leaves.

4. Wrap with wide gauze to hold compress in place. Elevate the injured joint. Repeat twice a day until swelling is gone.

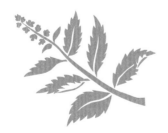

WARTS

What they are: Visually, warts are small, hard, white or pink lumps known as benign skin tumors that are caused by a family of viruses called papillomavirus. The common wart typically appears on the hand but can occur on other parts of the body.

Wart viruses are spread by touch. The virus must come in contact with the skin (even a handshake). If there is a small break or tear in the skin, the virus will have access to deeper, living cells that can then be infected. During the period of damage, the virus will stimulate skin cells to grow and divide, producing the small, visible, warty lesions.

Anyone can have warts. They are most common in teenagers and adults under thirty. Those with suppressed immune systems may be more susceptible.

Distinguishing Warts and Moles

Warts and moles have different appearances. Common warts are hard lumps with a cauliflower-like surface and tiny black flecks that are really the ends of blood vessels. Plantar warts are so named because they appear on the soles of the feet. They are flattened by the pressure of walking. Moles are usually small circles of dark, pigmented skin that can occur anywhere on the body. A mole may be flat or raised and sometimes has hairs growing from it.

Warts are transmitted by viruses. Moles can be present from birth and some may develop during childhood.

Generally, warts are a nuisance but are not dangerous. However, if a mole changes in appearance, a physician should check it for the possibility that it has become malignant. It then may need to be removed.

Suggested remedies: Fifty percent of all warts will disappear without treatment. Seventy percent that are surgically or chemically removed stay away. The rest are a continual nuisance. Scratching and picking at warts spreads them by bringing existing viruses to the surface; scratching also stimulates the mother wart to enlarge and thicken. If you suffer from warts, try applications of any of the following natural remedies.

Greater celandine juice: Put a few drops of the fresh, orange-yellow juice from the stem of the greater celandine plant directly on the wart. Allow the juice to dry and remain on the spot for as long as possible. Repeat daily until the wart begins to disappear. It can be a slow process but it is usually successful. Discontinue if there is any unusual burning sensation. *Caution:* Do not use this herb if you are pregnant. Don't use celandine on the face or on large clusters of warts.

Willow bark: James Duke, Ph.D., author of *The Green Pharmacy,* suggests taping a small, moistened piece of the inner bark of a willow tree to the wart. Apply a new piece of inner bark daily for five to seven days.

KISS THE PRINCE

Shortly before her wedding, my friend's daughter, Karen, came to me with the problem of warts. At that time, I had not used celandine as a treatment but had heard of its long folk usage. Karen and her fiancé had purchased a home and invited me to visit. Their house faced on a small wooded lot and the previous owners had been away for a while. As I walked up the front steps, there, growing in the cracks, was *Chelidonium majus* itself. I began to think that there is no such thing as a coincidence.

Karen was willing to try an experiment with the caveat that if there was any discomfort, she would immediately rinse off the liquid. Every day, she dabbed the brightly colored celandine stem juice on her warts. The warts began to shrink and were completely gone in time for the wedding. This trial does not a research study make, but it is folk history repeating itself.

PART III:
SOOTHING FOOT CARE

Herbal Treatments, Massage,
and Exercises for Healthy Feet

Stephanie L. Tourles

INTRODUCTION
The Humble Foot

Anywhere you look or listen, be it magazines, television, radio, retail stores, or mail-order catalogues, you're bombarded with beauty industry media revolving around hair, skin, and nail care; diet and exercise programs; thinner thigh and anti-cellulite creams; hair color to restore your lost youth; or promises of whiter and brighter teeth in seven days. The humble foot is an often ignored body part. Products for the feet make up a very small percentage of sales in the health and beauty segment of the market. Why?

I have an inkling that one reason is because the foot is one of the least–seen parts of the body. It's not glamorous, it rarely gets shown off, so it doesn't receive the attention that other body parts do: The foot doesn't get styled, brushed, or buffed, and it doesn't need whitening or slimming. It's not used for attracting a mate (unless, that is, your mate of choice has a foot fetish). The foot is usually not exposed to the public, except during the summer months, when many people would rather hide their feet than showcase them. I've never even heard of a contest for the most beautiful feet, have you? I bet even beauty queens don't have beautiful feet — especially after forcing them into uncomfortable, 3-inch heels for hours, perhaps days, on end.

The average person's foot is just plain unattractive and taken for granted. Maybe you occasionally use a pumice stone to grind down your calluses, cut your toenails, massage lotion into your heels, or possibly even paint your nails. But the majority of the time you ignore your feet and simply stuff them, day after day, into ill-fitting shoes and expect them to feel just peachy!

There's actually very little literature about foot care available to the public, unless you know where to look or have an interest. But I hope to change that with this text. In it you will find topics on everything from nutrition for healthy feet to medical problems and their solutions, to advice on proper footwear, professional and home pedicures, and massage. I hope it will be an eye-opening book for you and make you think twice about your "dogs" and begin to appreciate them. Foot care shouldn't be a chore. With all the recipes in this book, you'll soon look forward to "feet treats" as a way of unwinding or of perking up.

I should mention that while I was doing research on the herbal foot care recipes presented here, I made and experimented with so many salves, lotions, creams, and scrubs that by the end of my creative period, I took notice of the condition of my skin and nails. Everything was positvely glowing — particularly my feet, which had been the focus of all that pampering. I had incredibly silky smooth skin everywhere; even my normally callused feet were soft. Getting into a daily habit of slathering yourself with beneficial, handmade herbal products really pays off!

I hope the recipes presented here appeal to you. Try as many recipes as you can. You'll have fun, learn a lot, and your feet will thank you.

—Stephanie L. Tourles

CHAPTER 7
Meet Your Feet: Foot Basics

▼▼▼▼

If your feet could speak, what would they say?

"We're so cramped in these tight, pointy shoes, we're nearly numb," say the fashionable woman's feet.

"These shoes smell so bad it's embarrassing," say the feet of a young athlete.

"Our toes are ugly and deformed, we've got corns everywhere, we ache, and you've painted our toenails a deep purple frost. Please don't show us in public!" say the feet of a hip young woman. (This is what my feet were saying in high school!)

"We can't breathe. Your designer Italian leather loafers and nylon socks are choking us. We look gorgeous but we're dying in here . . . please give us some air!" say the style-conscious attorney's feet.

If your feet could speak, they'd probably complain, and loudly. Our feet allow us to run, walk, jump, and skip, taking us where we need to go, often with grace and style. It's very difficult to get along without them. So what do we do to keep them in tip-top shape? Abuse them!

You're going to hear me say this over and over again throughout this section: Ill-fitting shoes are the source of most foot problems. We stuff our feet into high heels or loafers with narrow toes or wrap them in nylon socks or stockings so they can't breathe. We buy shoes that are too small or inflexible and that irritate our feet. We also tend to wear shoes long past their designated life span until all the supportive cushioning is no longer able to do its job.

In addition to shoe abuse, our feet also suffer from lack of daily hygiene. How many people actually wash and scrub their feet (including the soles and between the toes), much less actually dry between the toes? When we bathe or shower most of us just assume that the soap and shampoo that runs onto our feet is sufficient. All of this neglect can lead to foot problems (see chapter 11, Common Foot Problems, Uncommon Remedies, for an alphabetical list of foot problems and their treatments).

Avoiding these problems starts with basic foot care, wearing appropriate shoes, and giving your feet the occasional pampering treatment, all of which I cover in later chapters. First, here are some basics on the structure and function of your feet.

YOUR AMAZING FOOT

A masterpiece of design, that's what your foot is. Your complex, small foot contains some 26 bones (both feet contain a quarter of the bones in your entire body), 33 joints, and 112 ligaments, and a complicated network of blood vessels, tendons, and nerves. All of these interworking parts enable you to move gracefully, with balance and speed if you so wish. The heel pad and arches of your foot act as shock absorbers, cushioning blows and jolts that occur with every step.

Basic daily living, doing your household chores, walking around your office or in the grocery store, or just walking the dog, exerts several hundred tons of pressure on your feet over the course of the day. Feet experience more wear and tear in a lifetime than any other body part, and thus are more prone to injury. Of all the physical ailments people have, foot problems may be the most common.

Foot shape, size, arch height, and length of toes vary from person to person. The feet you have are an inherited combination from your parents, which may predispose you to several foot problems, including bunions, high arches, or Morton's foot.

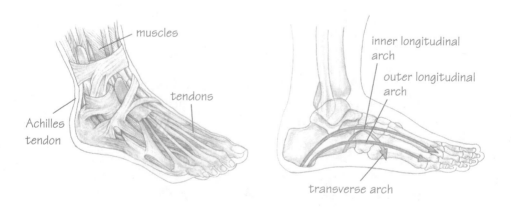

muscles

tendons

Achilles tendon

inner longitudinal arch

outer longitudinal arch

transverse arch

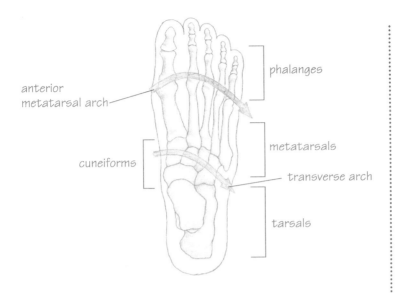

phalanges

anterior
metatarsal arch

cuneiforms

metatarsals

transverse arch

tarsals

Toenails

Toenails are composed of the same protein as your skin and hair, keratin. They just happen to have a harder composition. Their purpose is to protect the ends of your toes and the bones and nerves lying underneath. Toenails grow approximately ¹⁄₁₆ inch to ⅛ inch (1.6 mm to 3 mm) per month, slower than fingernails.

Your toenails can suffer a variety of disorders caused by injury, poor hygiene, poor circulation, or disease, such as bruises, tears, thick nails, ingrown nails, fungus, club nail, discoloration, brittleness, and curved growth. The elderly are especially susceptable to toenail problems due to failing eyesight and lack of strength to properly cut their nails, or simply because they can't bend over to do proper maintenance.

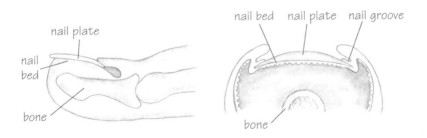

nail plate

nail
bed

bone

nail bed   nail plate   nail groove

bone

FOOT CARE BASICS

Treat your feet with tender loving care and they'll reward you with years of diligent, pain-free service. Just follow these simple guidelines for healthy, happy feet.

◆ Wash your feet daily. Make sure to get between the toes and under the nails.

◆ Completely dry your feet after bathing. Make sure to get between the toes when drying, too. Damp feet provide a breeding ground for bacteria and odor.

◆ To help prevent dry, cracked foot skin, massage a good thick lotion into your feet before you dress and again before you go to bed.

◆ Add a little foot powder to your shoes each day to help absorb perspiration.

◆ Wear fresh socks or hosiery daily.

◆ Cut your toenails straight across to help avoid ingrown toenails. Afterwards, smooth nail edges with an emery board or nail file.

◆ Inspect your feet daily for blisters, corns, calluses, swelling or other problems and treat accordingly. An ounce of prevention is worth a pound of cure.

◆ Give your shoes a rest. Alternating pairs allows shoes to completely dry out and gives the padding time to return to its normal shape. This makes shoes last longer and keeps your feet healthier.

◆ Give yourself a weekly "feet treat." Massage your feet with warmed oil mixed with a few drops of essential oil of lavender, eucalyptus, or peppermint to de-stress and relax your sore feet. I can hear them now: "Ahhhhh, that feels good!"

◆ If you're overweight, lose some pounds. Excess weight adds enormous pressure to your already stressed feet.

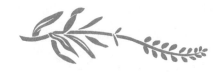

SUPPLIES: BANDAGING AND CUSHIONING AGENTS

Feet take a lot of abuse from tight, ill-fitting shoes, excessive exercise, or injuries from going barefoot. Sometimes genetics causes us to be predisposed to certain foot problems that can get worse with age. Occasionally our feet need a little cushioning, support, and tender loving care.

Podiatrists and orthopaedists often recommend to their patients various types of bandaging and cushioning materials to treat minor foot problems at home and help prevent them from developing further. All of the following products are available at finer retail and sporting goods outlets, drugstores or pharmacies, and supermarkets.

ADHESIVE TAPE (POROUS AND NONPOROUS)
Description: A white or beige tape that comes in ½-, 1-, 2-, and 3-inch widths.
Uses: Used to hold bandages on an injured foot or ankle. Frequently used as a secure wrap to support weak ankles, arches, and sore heels. The ½-inch strips can hold a corn pad in place and also cover the portion of your foot that is blister prone. Use the porous tape if the area you are covering needs to breathe (e.g., blisters, cuts, etc.) Note: This tape does not stretch, so it will not always stay in place during activity.

ADHESIVE FELT
Description: Thicker than moleskin with soft felt on one side and adhesive on the other.
Uses: Can be cut into any shape to form custom padding for corns, sore callused areas, blisters, bunions, and metatarsal and heel pain.

CORN PADS
Description: Round or oval felt or moleskin pads. Available with or without adhesive. Can be custom made by cutting your own out of a larger piece of adhesive felt or moleskin.

> **FOOT FACT**
>
> Corns mostly affect women, who often wear tight, ill-fitting, or high-heeled shoes. Nine percent of women get corns annually.

Uses: These pads put a cushion of protection between your sensitive corn and your shoe, relieving the friction or pressure between the two. The corn will then gradually disappear.

ELASTICIZED ADHESIVE TAPE

Description: The same as regular adhesive tape, but stretches and gives with body movement.

Uses: Good for active people because it stretches with foot movement and will hold any added padding and protective cushioning in place. Also, if you get it wet, it will dry and retain its shape. Elasticized tape won't tend to fall off like regular adhesive tape.

GAUZE

Description: An all-purpose foot treatment material, gauze is basically folded cheesecloth. It is usually sold in sterile, packaged squares. Because it is porous, gauze allows whatever is beneath to breathe.

Uses: To cover blister-prone areas and prevent shoes from rubbing you the wrong way. It is also useful for covering any minor injuries to your foot. Gauze should be held in place with elastic or regular adhesive tape, depending on your needs.

GEL PADS

Description: Gel-filled, plastic pads that come in many shapes and sizes. Some are designed specifically as cushioning devices for the heel or ball of the foot. They are also available as full-length cushioning inserts.

Uses: These provide a soothing layer of comfort cushioning between you and your hard shoes. Not recommended for high heels.

HEEL CUP

Description: Made of plastic or rubber and worn inside the shoe to fit snugly around the bottom and sides of the heel.

Uses: Provides thick cushioning and proper heel support to help alleviate plantar fasciitis (heel pain) and the pain of heel spurs. Absorbs and disperses the shock when your heel strikes the ground.

HEEL PADS

Description: Made of foam rubber or foam rubber covered with plastic to cover the bottom of the heel.

Uses: Used to cushion a sore heel. Can be customized into any shape, such as cutting a hole where a heel spur or bruise is so there is cushioning all around the sore spot and the pressure is relieved on the painful area.

INSOLES

Description: Insoles are generally three-quarter-length or full-length padded shoe inserts. They are available in many versions: foam rubber, gel-filled, terry cloth lined, arch support, athletic support, and odor-destroyers with baking soda.

Uses: There's an insole designed for just about every shoe whether you wear high heels, sneakers, or steel-toed construction boots. They provide added cushioning just where you need it most.

LAMB'S WOOL

Description: Silky, smooth, white lamb's wool. It feels very soft, like kitten fur.

Uses: This product feels like silk against your skin. It's great to use on blisters or corns between your toes or to wrap around a toe if you have a blister or sore callus on top. A piece of lamb's wool can also be taped in place if you have a "hot spot" on your heel that is about to blister.

MOLESKIN

Description: Moleskin is thinner than adhesive felt. Cushioned on one side and adhesive on the other, it comes in rectangular sheets. Did they derive the name from the softness of a mole's pelt? My cats have brought me plenty and believe me, they're the softest little critters I've ever felt!

Uses: Can use the same way as adhesive felt (see above).

TOOLS OF THE FOOT TRADE: EQUIPMENT FOR HERBAL FOOT CARE PRODUCTS

You probably already own all of the kitchen gadgets required to make, use, and store your personalized foot care products, with the exception of a few storage containers. I haven't asked you to purchase anything exotic or expensive, except for the food processor, which is handy but not an absolute necessity.

I am a real stickler about two things when it comes to being a kitchen cosmetologist. First, everything you use must be sterile. If it's impractical to boil the tool or storage container, then run it through the dishwasher or soak it in very, very hot soapy water for fifteen minutes and give it a good scrub. You don't want to encourage bacterial growth in your products.

Second, never use aluminum or copper pans or bowls when making lotions, salves, creams, liniments, or tinctures. These metals can react with the herb and acid liquids in your recipes and leach the aluminum or copper into the foot care formula you're making. At the very least, they can discolor the end product.

Large Equipment

These kitchen tools can range in price from approximately $20 to $175 or so. The fancier, more heavy duty, or more high tech, the more expensive. Don't buy cheap tools; they'll only wear out quickly and have to be replaced, which means they weren't so cheap after all! Middle-of-the-road quality is fine, unless you love to indulge yourself and always buy top of the line.

BLENDER
I use this for making creams and lotions in 1 cup (230 ml) quantities or more. With smaller quantities I have difficulty extracting the product from the bottom. You can also use it to grind oatmeal, nuts, seeds, and herbs, but a coffee grinder does a much better job.

COFFEE GRINDER
This is one of my most used kitchen gadgets. It is the same as a nut/seed grinder. I grind oatmeal, almonds, and beans into powders for facial, body, and foot scrubs. Larger and harder herb

pieces can be ground into much finer pieces, though not always into baby-fine powder. Note: Don't grind herbs in the same coffee grinder that you grind coffee beans in, or the coffee will have a "wangy" taste and the herbs will smell and taste of coffee!

FOOD PROCESSOR

This can replace the blender and do some nut grinder chores too. Great for thoroughly mixing up a *large* batch of lotion (2 cups or more), foot scrub, or powder.

POTS AND PANS

Use stainless steel, glass, or enamel only, please. It's best to have a variety of sizes, including a 1-pint (460 ml) saucepan and 1-, 2-, 3-, and 6-quart (1-, 2-, 3-, and 6-liter) pots. I use all sizes for melting oils and beeswax to make lotions, creams, and salves, and for boiling water for herbal foot bath teas, and extracting gelatinous substances from herb roots.

Small Tools

These are basic items that make your life simpler. You probably have many of these items in your kitchen. Creating products at home, especially creams, lotions, and salves, sometimes requires a lot of stirring. When choosing stirring devices, try to get instruments that you're comfortable with and that fit into your hand nicely.

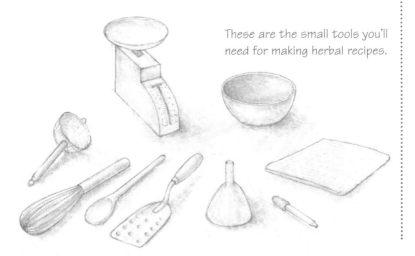

These are the small tools you'll need for making herbal recipes.

BOWLS

From small to large, glass, plastic, enamel, or stainless steel, all come in handy for one recipe or another. I use larger ones for mixing foot scrubs and powders in quantity (usually for gifts) and small ones for single-use or small batches of massage oils, foot scrubs, and foot spray mixtures.

CHEESECLOTH OR HOSIERY

These are for keeping herbal foot bath mixtures from getting in your foot tub. Just place your ingredients into the cheesecloth or hosiery, tie up with string, and let it float about, releasing the beneficial properties while keeping your foot tub tidy. They also make great strainers for herb teas and salves. The hosiery does the best job of screening out fine particulate matter.

EYEDROPPERS

Try to have several glass ones on hand. I use these only as a measuring device for essential oils. Some bottles of essential oils come with their own dropper, but over time the rubber at the end of the dropper will soften and allow air to enter the oils and cause their healing properties to diminish. Always sterilize before use.

FUNNEL

A small funnel comes in handy when pouring herbal recipes into narrow-necked storage bottles. Aluminum foil can be fashioned into a funnel in a snap. No need to worry about the aluminum in this case, because the liquid is in such brief contact with the foil that there's no danger of any metal leaching into the product.

MEASURING CUPS AND SPOONS

You probably have plenty of these standard items for measuring and stirring your herbal concoctions. If not, garage sales and flea markets are good places to buy extras.

SCALE

A tabletop or diet scale is not a necessity, but it's nice to have if you like to know how much your final product weighs. In this section, I don't use ounces as measurements in my recipes, so you can get away without purchasing one. It can be eye-opening to see that 4 ounces (112 g) of German chamomile flowers takes up quite a lot of space versus 4 ounces (112 g) of powdered marshmallow root! It's a nice piece of equipment to have around.

SPATULA

For scraping creams and lotions from blenders and food processors or any type of container, these tools in small and medium sizes are wonderful. I use both narrow and wide blade types. These are also handy for whipping creams, lotions, and salves using the same wrist action you use to beat frosting or egg whites.

STRAINER

When straining herb teas, liniments, and salve mixtures that have large herb matter, I use a mesh strainer. When I need to strain more finely ground herbs, I line it with cheesecloth or pantyhose.

WHISKS

I like to use a large whisk to gently blend large batches of foot and body powder. Whisks mix the herbs and essential oils evenly. Small whisks are super for whipping small quantities of creams, lotions, and salves. I find whisks with a fat handle easier and more comfortable to hold than those with skinny handles.

WOODEN SPOONS

These can be used to stir anything. They are especially good if you're making herbal vinegar–based remedies. The wood won't react with the acid as a metal spoon or whisk might.

Storage Containers

When you make herbal foot care products, you've got to have something to store them in, plain and simple. Choose a container that's aesthetically pleasing and is the appropriate container for the product. See Resources, or look at antique sales and flea markets for old ornamental boxes, bottles, jars, and tins.

BOTTLES

You'll need a variety of these, both plastic and glass, in sizes from 2 to 16 ounces (55 to 454 g). Plastic, narrow-necked bottles with or without a squirt top are the obvious choice for anyone concerned about breakage or someone who travels a lot.

I prefer to use dark cobalt blue, green, or amber glass bottles when I can for two reasons: One, they're pretty (I like the old-fashioned apothecary look); two, the dark-colored glass helps preserve the volatile oils of the herbs and essential oils inside. Make sure the bottles you choose have tight-fitting tops.

JARS

Widemouthed canning jars, ½ pint-, pint-, and quart-sized (230 ml, 460 ml, and 1 l) are perfect for making infused herbal oils, liniments, and tinctures. Use screw-top glass or plastic jars in sizes from 1 to 4 ounces (28 to 112 g) for storing foot scrubs, salves, and creams.

SHAKER JAR

Plastic culinary herb containers from the grocery store can be recycled and used for your powders. The inner top is usually full of holes, perfect for dispensing herb powders. Glass containers are harder to find, but nice to have. Cardboard cylinder shakers are usually sold through herbal mail-order suppliers.

SPRITZER

A must-have for your cooling foot sprays, spritzers are available in 1-, 2-, 4-, and 8-ounce (28-, 55-, 112-, and 228-gram) glass or plastic bottles. Hair spray bottles can be recycled for this purpose.

TINS

Tins have a lovely old-fashioned appeal and look very attractive if decorated with a custom-made label. I like to use these to store dried herbs, foot and body powders with a puff, and dry foot and body scrubs. Tins are available in sizes from ¼ ounce to 8 ounces (7 to 228 g) and larger and sold in better hardware, herb stores, and through mail order.

TOOLS AT A GLANCE

Blender
Bottles
Bowls
Cheesecloth or hosiery
Coffee grinder (nut/seed grinder)
Eyedropper
Food processor
Funnel
Jars
Measuring cups and spoons
Pots and pans
Scale
Shakers
Spatula
Spritzer
Strainer
Tins
Whisks
Wooden spoons

CHAPTER 8
Home Pedicure

Granted, a home pedicure isn't as luxurious as a professional one, but it is a wonderful way to give yourself a little TLC. It's beautification and relaxation rolled into one treatment.

Even if I've had an absolutely awful day at work and I am emotionally drained, just knowing that my hands and feet are well manicured and looking spectacular gives me the feeling (even though it's superficial) that I do still have the upper hand, that there is a bit of order in this chaotic life of mine. You might be surprised to find that I'm not the only person to think this way. We are many!

A pedicure makes your feet look and feel great.

I give myself various foot treatments several times a week. I use a salt and extra-virgin olive oil foot scrub once a week, file my callused areas with a pediwand two to three times per week, trim and/or file my toenails once a week, massage in a thick foot cream twice a week for a night treatment, and use a foot and face mask at the same time once a week to soften and remove dead skin. I have high-maintenance feet and they need the care, but I also *enjoy* "fussing" (as my husband calls it) or "pampering" (as I call it), and taking good care of myself.

PROFESSIONAL TIPS
TO KEEP FEET IN SUPER SHAPE

- Use a good sloughing lotion two to three times per week to keep dry, flaky skin at bay.
- Smooth your calluses with a good foot file or rasp one to two times per week.
- Inspect toenails once a week and trim and shape as necessary.
- Have a professional pedicure once a month if possible.
- Walk, walk, walk, walk. . . .

Consistent and proper care of anything — be it your face, hair, hands, or feet — pays high dividends in the long run. You'll stay more youthful-looking longer and be more comfortable to boot!

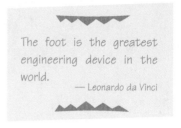

The foot is the greatest engineering device in the world.
— Leonardo da Vinci

EQUIPMENT NEEDED

Here's a list of the basic items you'll need to give your feet the royal treatment. I'm sure you have most of them in your bathroom and you can make the others from my recipes.

- ◆ **Foot tub.** It's a good idea to have two of these, so one can be used as a rinsing bath. They should be big enough so you can swish your feet around a bit. The simplest are large plastic tubs, but you can get fancy and buy a vibrating whirlpool footbath.
- ◆ **Towels.** Have two of these ready also, one to use underneath the foot tub to catch drips and one for drying your feet.
- ◆ **Comfortable chair**
- ◆ **Toenail clippers**
- ◆ **Emery board.** Use this to file nails and pare down corns.
- ◆ **Pediwand, pumice foot rasp, or pumice stone.** These three implements do basically the same thing. They give you a real edge when it comes to removing callused and rough skin. The pediwand and rasp are shaped the same, except that the pediwand has coarse sandpaper on one side and fine on the other, and the rasp has an oval pumice stone attached to it. I prefer either of these to a stone because they're much easier to hold.

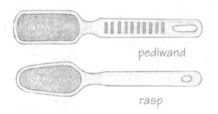

pediwand

rasp

pumice stones

- **Orange stick.** Used for pushing back cuticles and removing debris under toenails.
- **Corn and callus trimmer.** This is actually a razor or series of razors with a handle. Used judiciously and with a steady hand, it will remove very thick, hard calluses and the tops of some hard corns. Many men use these when sloughing creams and pediwands just aren't abrasive enough. Be *extremely careful* not to cut too deep and draw blood. **Caution:** Diabetics should never use this tool.

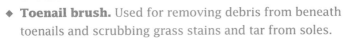

corn and callus trimmer

- **Toenail brush.** Used for removing debris from beneath toenails and scrubbing grass stains and tar from soles.
- **Essential oils.** Invigorating oils: camphor, eucalyptus, any mint, tea tree, juniper, bergamot, rosemary, clove, lemon, or orange. Relaxing oils: lavender, geranium, German chamomile, rose, clary sage, almond, or vanilla. You'll need one or more of these to put in your foot bath, foot scrub, cream, and powder.
- **Foot powder.** Serves to freshen, fragrance, and deodorize feet. Try the Flower Powder recipe on the next page.
- **Nail polish, nonacetone polish remover, and cotton balls.**
- **Foot scrub.** Try my Autumn Spice Skin Exfoliator recipe on page 159.
- **Foot cream.** Use this as a massage cream during your pedicure and as a daily softening foot treatment cream. Try making the Lavender Velvet Cream recipe on page 160.

SANITATION OF EQUIPMENT

Your personal pedicure tools should be thoroughly cleansed and scrubbed in hot soapy water, then rinsed with 90 percent isopropyl rubbing alcohol approximately twice a month. If someone in your home has contagious athlete's foot, plantar warts, or toenail fungus, they should have their own set of tools and thoroughly disinfect them as well as their hands and any towels used immediately after performing a pedicure to avoid spreading the disease to other family members. To be on the safe side, the infected family member should store his or her tools in a separate place.

FLOWER POWDER

¼ cup (60 ml) fine, white cosmetic clay

¼ cup (60 ml) corn-starch

2 tablespoons (30 ml) finely ground and sifted dried lavender flowers

2 tablespoons (30 ml) finely ground and sifted dried rose petals

2 tablespoons (30 ml) finely ground and sifted dried chamomile flowers

10 drops orange essential oil

10 drops lavender essential oil

10 drops rose or geranium essential oil

Yield: approximately ¾ cup (180 ml)

To make: Combine all ingredients in a medium-sized bowl.

To use: Sprinkle liberally on feet and legs after pedicure, sprinkle daily in your shoes, or use as a body powder.

Optional: Men can create a more masculine fragrance by omitting the floral herbs and oils and substituting 1 teaspoon (5 ml) cinnamon powder, 1 teaspoon powdered cloves, 1 teaspoon powdered allspice or nutmeg, and 30 drops orange, lemon, or lime essential oil.

Storage: Store in a shaker container or a small box with a puff in a cool, dry place.

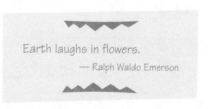

Earth laughs in flowers.

— Ralph Waldo Emerson

AUTUMN SPICE SKIN EXFOLIATOR

Here's a fragrant recipe with which to treat your feet. It's great for smoothing out the rough spots on your feet and legs.

1/2 cup (125 ml) ground oatmeal

2 tablespoons (30 ml) ground almonds or sunflower seeds

1 tablespoon (15 ml) cornmeal

1 tablespoon (15 ml) sea salt

1 tablespoon (15 ml) powdered nutmeg

1 tablespoon (15 ml) powdered allspice

1 tablespoon (15 ml) powdered cloves

1 tablespoon (15 ml) finely ground, dried orange peel

15 drops orange essential oil

10 drops geranium essential oil

5 drops clove essential oil

Yield: approximately 1 cup (250 ml)

To make:

1. Grind the oatmeal and the almonds in a nut/seed grinder or coffee grinder until they are the consistency of coarse parmesan cheese.

2. In a small plastic storage container, mix all recipe ingredients thoroughly.

To use:

1. In a small bowl, combine approximately 2 tablespoons (30 ml) of dry mix with 2 tablespoons (30 ml) (more or less) orange juice, milk, rosewater, or plain water until a spreadable paste forms. The amount of liquid you use will depend on how finely ground your herbs and seeds are. Add liquid a little at a time until you get the perfect consistency. The mixture will continue to thicken if you let it stand for a few minutes.

2. Massage onto dry lower legs and feet in circular motions, making sure to get in between toes. Do this for as long as you desire, but at least 5 minutes total, and then rinse. Leaves skin smooth as silk and delightfully scented, too.

Storage: Store dry ingredients for up to one year in tightly sealed plastic storage container away from light and moisture.

LAVENDER VELVET CREAM

This scented cream is a great daily foot treatment. It's one of my favorites.

½ cup (125 ml) all-vegetable shortening

1 teaspoon (5 ml) beeswax

3 tablespoons (45 ml) distilled water, rose water, German chamomile tea, or lavender tea

1 teaspoon (5 ml) borax

15 drops lavender essential oil

15 drops rose or geranium essential oil

5 drops spearmint essential oil (optional, but adds a nice, mild minty note)

Yield: approximately ¾ cup (180 ml)

To make:

1. In a small saucepan, heat the shortening and beeswax over very low heat until just melted. Remove saucepan from heat.

2. In another small saucepan, warm the distilled water and dissolve the borax in it; then remove saucepan from heat. (To make an herb tea to use as your liquid, simply pour 1 cup [230 ml] boiling water over 1 teaspoon [5 ml] of dried herb, steep 5 to 10 minutes, then strain.)

3. When both mixtures have cooled to approximately the same temperature, set the wax/shortening pan into a bowl of ice cubes and add the essential oils.

4. Drizzle the liquid into it, stirring rapidly with a small whisk or spoon. The cream should set up fairly quickly and look and feel like fluffy cake icing.

To use: Slather it thickly onto clean feet, put on socks, and go to bed. Awaken to "feet of velvet." This product can be used wherever you have dry skin: hands, elbows, knees, or even as a cuticle conditioner. It sinks in amazingly fast, is non-greasy if you don't use too much, and makes your skin super soft.

Storage: Store in an attractive container away from heat or light. No need to refrigerate unless weather is hot. Will last approximately one year if you do choose to chill it or up to three to four months at room temperature.

DO-IT-YOURSELF PEDICURE PROCEDURE

Set aside about an hour one evening per week to treat your feet. Surround yourself with all of the necessary supplies so you don't have to keep getting up and dripping water all over the house.

Step 1: A good soak. A footbath is often just as relaxing or stimulating as a full-body bath. The feet are one of the most receptive parts of the body. To your foot tub, add enough hot or cold water or herbal tea of choice to cover your ankles plus a few drops of tea tree essential oil or one tablespoon (15 ml) of bleach to disinfect and a squirt of liquid soap or shower gel. Swish them together. Soak your feet for five to ten minutes to cleanse and soften calluses. Use this time to scrub dirty toenails and soles, too.

Step 2: After soaking, gently remove calluses with a pedi-wand, rasp, stone, or if you must, very carefully use a callus trimmer. File any corns down with an emery board.

Step 3: Dry feet and legs when finished and remove any old, chipped nail polish now.

Step 4: Try my Autumn Spice Skin Exfoliator (see recipe on page 159) to scrub off any leftover rough skin on your lower legs, ankles, and feet. It feels fantastic and smells great, too!

If you're short on time (and who isn't) whip up the Peppermint Salt Glo exfoliating recipe (see box) instead.

PEPPERMINT SALT GLO

1 tablespoon (15 ml) sea salt
1 tablespoon (15 ml) extra-virgin olive oil
5 drops peppermint essential oil

Yield: 1 treatment
To make: In a small bowl, combine all ingredients, stirring thoroughly.
To use: Massage onto lower legs, ankles, and feet, using a circular motion. Aim for 3 to 5 minutes on each leg and foot. It feels quite invigorating and refreshing and is great to use on a hot summer day!

Step 5: Rinse. Then dry legs and feet with a coarse towel.

Step 6: Coax back cuticles with an orange stick and trim any that are ragged.

Step 7: Trim toenails straight across rather than rounded at the corners so that the white free edge is almost even with the top of the toe. File toenails to smooth any jagged edges.

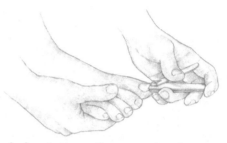

Step 8: Apply foot lotion, oil, or cream and massage in thoroughly for two to three minutes on each foot. Follow the steps in chapter 10, page 174, if you wish.

Step 9: If polishing your toenails, apply a nonacetone remover now to remove all traces of lotion or cream. Now slick on a base coat and two coats of your favorite color, followed by a top coat. There's nothing like ten freshly painted, glossy, perfectly pedicured toes to pick you up and make you feel pretty!

Step 10: After your polish dries, apply your favorite powder to your legs and feet using a large puff or fluff brush to fragrance and prevent perspiration from taking a foothold.

I have two other foot care recipes I'd like to share with you that can be included in your weekly pedicure to add a little variety.

OPTIONAL TOOL FOR DRY LEGS AND FEET

A loofah sponge or coconut fiber brush is wonderful for dry-brushing your legs and feet upon arising each morning and for revving up circulation. If you tend to be plagued with dry skin, a daily brushing starting with your feet and working up to your thighs will quickly banish your scaly skin problem. Remember to wash and dry this tool once a week.

ANTIBACTERIAL FOOT SOAP

1 8-ounce (224-gram) bottle liquid castile soap (Available in health food stores or from mail-order suppliers. I prefer peppermint scent, but almond is nice, too.)

10 drops tea tree essential oil

10 drops thyme essential oil

Yield: 8 ounces (224 grams)

To make: Add essential oils to bottle and shake well.

To use: Add a squirt or two to footbath to help clean and disinfect feet and kill bacteria and fungus.

Storage: Will keep in a squirt bottle up to one year.

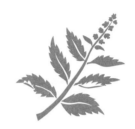

STEP LIVELY SLOUGHING FOOT MASK

The clay in this recipe acts as an astringent, drawing impurities from the feet, and it stimulates circulation and removes dry skin. The apple or grape juice contains natural alpha-hydroxy acids, which also slough and soften skin. It's good for feet suffering from poison ivy, insect bites, eczema, or psoriasis.

3 tablespoons (45 ml) green clay or bentonite clay

Enough water, apple, or grape juice to form a paste (fresh-pressed juices are best)

Yield: 1 treatment

To make: Combine ingredients in a small bowl, stirring until a smooth paste is formed.

To use:

1. Apply clay in a medium-thick layer to clean, dry feet, covering them from the soles to the ankles. Allow to dry for 30 minutes.

2. Rinse, then dry with coarse towel.

3. Apply thick cream and cover with socks overnight.

CHAPTER 9
Exercises for the Feet

$\blacktriangledown\blacktriangledown\blacktriangledown\blacktriangledown$

Think back . . . way back. How did you arrive into this world? Were you born with shoes on? Tight socks or hosiery? Did you have corns, calluses, hammertoes, or bunions? No! You arrived buck naked, soft, smooth, and *barefoot.*

In a world void of concrete, asphalt, tar, broken glass, metal, chewing gum, hot pavement, corporate dress codes, or fashion trends, you could continue to go through life barefoot and carefree, or at the very most wear loose sandals in summer and warm, loose moccasins in the winter (some people do). But, alas, most of us do not live in such a place.

For the shoe-wearing masses, specific foot exercises can be of great benefit to strengthen and stretch the muscles of the foot, relieve cramping and strain in the arches, ease heel pain, and the pain of hammertoes, bunions, and toe cramps. Basically, foot exercises can help to counteract the symptoms of footwear abuse.

Some of you may wonder why you need to exercise your feet. You walk a little or a lot during each day, depending on your lifestyle, and that should be sufficient, right? Wrong! This walking that you routinely do is *probably* done in ill-fitting shoes. Even if you wear correct shoes you are still subjecting your feet to some type of rubbing, binding, pressure, or suffocation from lack of air circulation. Your feet, just like the rest of your body, need to be toned and stretched in their natural, unbound state: barefoot. You don't wear your work clothes to run, walk, or go to the gym, do you? You wear something loose and comfortable. So why would you wear shoes when you exercise your feet? Feet should be free and unfettered for at least ten hours per day. If you want your feet to provide you with years of uninterrupted service, treat them with the utmost care. Daily hygiene and a few exercises go a long way toward this goal. Do keep in mind though, that ten to fifteen minutes of foot exercise every day will *not* do any good if you continue to wear ill-fitting shoes that constrict movement and force your feet into unnatural shapes.

THE EXERCISES

The following foot, ankle, and toe exercises can be performed at any time you feel the need to stretch and release tension. If you can't slip off your shoes discreetly during the day, then perform the exercises when you get home from work or finish your daily errands. Slip your body into something more comfortable and slip your feet out of something uncomfortable (your shoes). Relax and unwind. A nice cup of soothing herbal tea, sipped while you do your exercises, tastes especially good, hot or cold!

Footsie Roller Massage

Wooden footsie rollers have been around for many years. They come in all shapes and sizes from single to double or triple rollers. Some are hand held and some sit on the floor. I particularly like the ones with raised ridges going from one end to the other. These are both stimulating and relaxing to my feet. My mother used to use this type when she massaged my feet as a teen. I'd fall asleep on the living room floor before she finished — it felt sooooo good!

If you don't have a footsie roller, a wooden rolling pin can be used in a pinch. Simply place the footsie roller or rolling pin on the floor and while bearing down comfortably, roll the entire length of your foot over the tool, back and forth, and back, concentrating on your arches. Do this for five to ten minutes per foot. This exercise relieves fatigue and cramping, especially in your arches.

FOOT REFRESHER AND DE-STRESSOR

This combined exercise and foot soak is designed to relax tired, aching feet, relieve toe cramps, and strengthen weak foot muscles that support the plantar fascia that runs the length of the bottom of your foot from the heel to the ball of the foot. This one is also good if you suffer from hammertoes and pain in the ball of your foot.

Foot tub

40–60 medium to large marbles

2 tablespoons (30 ml) yarrow or sage

2 tablespoons (30 ml) wintergreen

5–10 drops lavender, camphor, peppermint, rosemary, or eucalyptus essential oil

½ cup (125 ml) sea salt, baking soda, or Epsom salts

Large towel

Yield: 1 treatment

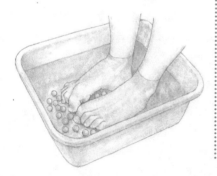

To make:

1. Place the foot tub with the marbles in it in front of a comfortable chair.

2. Boil enough water to fill the foot tub to above ankle height.

3. Remove water from heat and add the yarrow or sage and the wintergreen tightly tied in cheesecloth. Cover and steep for 15 minutes. Remove the herbs. (You can add the spent herbs to your compost pile.)

4. Fill the foot tub with the hot tea, and add the essential oil and the sea salt, baking soda, or Epsom salts. Swish the ingredients around to dissolve the salt and blend in essential oil.

To use:

1. Place your feet in the tub and roll them around on the marbles.

2. Pick up and release marbles with your toes, grasping marbles tightly, squeezing your toes, then releasing. Do this for 10 to 15 minutes.

3. Dry feet roughly with towel.

4. Slather with a thick moisturizer and put on socks.

RELAXING FOOT MASSAGE OIL

After washing and exercising your feet, use this fabulous aromatherapy herbal oil to further enhance your relaxed mode and soften any rough skin as well.

2 teaspoons (10 ml) soy-bean, jojoba, extra-virgin olive, or almond oil
2–6 drops (depending on strength desired) lavender, German chamomile, orange, or clary sage essential oil

Yield: 1 treatment

To make: Mix all ingredients thoroughly in a small bowl.
To use: Massage into feet using a firm, strong hand. Apply pressure as needed to alleviate fatigue and tension in your feet. Put on socks afterward. You may be ready to climb into bed at this point!

The Golf Ball Roll

This exercise is recommended by Carol Frey, M.D., Director of the Orthopaedic Foot and Ankle Center in Manhattan Beach, California. "Roll a golf ball under the ball of your foot for two minutes. This is great massage for the bottom of the foot and is recommended for people with plantar fasciitis (heel pain), arch strain, or foot cramps."

Point and Flex

This is a great exercise to stretch and strengthen just about everything from your knees down. Sit on the floor, legs stretched out in front of you and palms facing down at your sides. Now point your toes as hard as you can, hold for five seconds, then bend your foot up and curl your toes back as hard as you can and hold for five seconds. Repeat a total of 10 times. If you experience cramping, this usually means that your muscles are weak and need conditioning. Cut back on your repetitions, and gradually work up to 10.

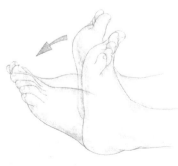

Heel Raises

Heel raises are especially good for women who wear high heels frequently. This shoe type stresses your arches, cramps your toes, and gradually shortens the Achilles tendon, which frequently leads to heel pain when you suddenly switch to a low-heeled shoe and stretch the shortened tendon. Heel raises strengthen your ankle, improve your balance, stretch the Achilles tendon, and provide overall foot conditioning.

This exercise can be performed using a 2-foot-long (60 cm) 6-by-6-inch block of wood or landscape timber or a thick telephone book, or it can be done on the bottom step of a set of stairs or on an exercise bench step. Whatever you use, make sure it's sturdy and won't tip over. Simply hang and lower your heels over the edge of the step, board, or book, as far as comfortably possible to give your heels and calves a good stretch. Now, raise up onto your toes. Go up and down for 20 to 30 repetitions.

An alternate exercise that requires a bit more balance and agility is called standing toe raises. This exercise is recommended by the American Orthopaedic Foot and Ankle Society. Simply "stand on one foot at a time and raise yourself slowly up onto your toes, then lower yourself back down." If your balance is a bit off, hang on to something with one hand to steady yourself. Work up to 20 to 30 repetitions with each foot.

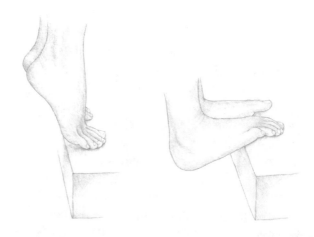

Runner's Stretch

Here's another stretching exercise for high heel wearers that's also good for athletes as a warm–up stretch for their lower leg muscles. It stretches the plantar fascia and Achilles tendon and is good for anyone suffering from heel pain.

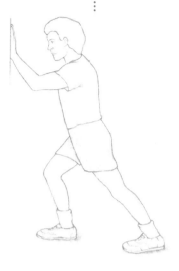

The runner's stretch is somewhat like doing a modified push-up against a wall. Stand approximately 3 feet (.9 m) away from a wall. With your right foot only, take one step about halfway toward the wall. Place palms against the wall at about shoulder height. As you slowly bend the right knee, lean into the wall while keeping both heels flat on the floor. Your left leg should be straight since this is the leg that is receiving the stretch. If you're doing it correctly, you will feel the back of your calf and the arch of your foot stretching. Hold this position for at least 10 seconds. Go back to the starting position, relax, and repeat 10 to 20 times. To exercise the right leg and foot, just reverse positions.

Ankle Strengthener

This particular movement strengthens ankles and helps to relieve stiffness in the ankle joint. It can be performed either by lying on your back and extending your legs up in the air or by sitting in a chair with one leg crossed over the other. I like to do these with a 1-pound (454 g) weight strapped around the middle of my foot. Wrist weights can also be used as long as they are not too tight for your foot. Weights are optional, of course.

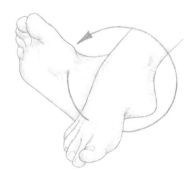

From either position, you simply draw circles with your feet 20 times each first in a clockwise, then counterclockwise, direction. This is a basic exercise, but it feels great at the end of a long day. It is very good as a morning warm-up exercise if you suffer from stiff, arthritic ankles.

Rubberband Big Toe Stretches

This exercise is helpful if you suffer from bunions or toe cramps resulting from wearing shoes with a narrow toe box and/or high heels. This exercise and the following one are also recommended by Carol Frey, M.D., Director of the Orthopaedic Foot and Ankle Center.

Either sit on the floor with your legs stretched out in front of you and your palms on the floor beside or behind you, or sit in a chair with your feet flat on the floor. Place a nice, thick, moderately stiff rubberband around your big toes and pull your feet away from each other. Hold for five to ten seconds, then relax. Repeat 10 to 20 times. If this hurts, or if you have arthritis or bunions in advanced stages, do only as many as you can and gradually increase as your toes gain strength.

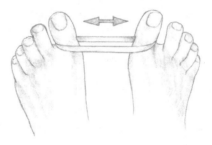

Toe Spreader

You may have seen those little pink foam toe separators used in salons to keep your freshly painted toenails from touching while they're drying. Well, you'll need that little device for this exercise.

Place the separator between your toes and squeeze your toes inward for five to ten seconds, then spread them for five to ten seconds. Relax. Repeat 10 times. This exercise is good for hammertoes, toe cramps, and forefoot pain due to wearing tight, ill-fitting shoes.

BENEFITS OF BAREFOOT WALKING

The best treatment for feet encased in shoes all day is to go bare-foot. One-fifth of the world's population never wear shoes — ever! But when people who usually go barefoot begin to wear shoes, their feet begin to suffer. As often as possible, walk barefoot on the beach, in your yard, or at least around the house. Walking in the grass or sand massages your feet, strengthens your muscles and feels very relax-ing. Caution: Please be very careful if you're diabetic. Walk only on clean surfaces to avoid cutting and puncturing your feet.

If you can cut back on wearing shoes by 30 percent, you will save wear and tear on your feet and extend the life of your shoes!

Arch Relief

The inner longitudinal arch, which is the arch that absorbs most of the shock of basic daily living, will feel stiff and ache from time to time. This exercise eases the tension and relaxes the muscles in this area.

To perform this exercise, walk on tip toe for thirty seconds, relax, then from a flat-footed stance, roll your feet outward so that you are standing on the outside edges of your feet and remain for fifteen seconds. Repeat 5 times.

Pencil Pick-Up

For those of you suffering from hammer-toes, pain in your forefoot, stiff ankles, or toe cramps, this exercise is for you. It also stretches the tendons on top of your foot. You will need 10 unsharpened pencils and a heavy mug. While sitting or standing, pick up one pencil at a time with your toes and place it into the mug. Repeat with the other foot.

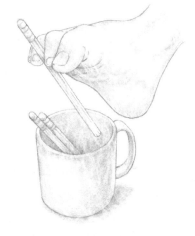

CHAPTER 10
Foot Massage:
Sweet Relief for Tired Feet

If your nerves are frayed, your energy level is running on empty, and your feet have seen better days, then by all means partake of an aromatherapy foot massage. It will soothe your spirits, reduce your stress, put the spring back into your step, and soften your feet. What's good for the body is good for the "sole"!

Take a good look at your feet after they've spent a day in snug leather shoes. What do they look like? Feel like? Do your toes look fresh and happy? Are your feet pink and healthy and rarin' to go and run about? Probably not. More than likely your ten toes are squished against each other, resembling sardines in a can. The skin of your feet looks lifeless, perhaps gray in color and slightly clammy to the touch. I don't think your feet are in the mood to respond positively to, "Tennis anyone?"

"If people bound and gagged the entire body the way they do their feet, none of us would live to the age of twenty," states Gordon Inkeles and Murray Todris, authors of *The Art of Sensual Massage.* If you think about it, they're probably right!

In the August 1997 issue of *Life* magazine, there appeared a wonderful article entitled, "The Magic of Touch: Massage's healing powers make it serious medicine," written by George H. Colt and Anne Hollister. Try to put your hands on a copy if you can. It's eye-opening! In it the authors state, "The idea that touch can heal is an old one. The first written records of massage (the word comes from an Arabic word meaning *stroke*) date back three thousand years to China. A bas-relief on the tomb of Ankh-mahor, an Egyptian priest who lived around 2200 B.C., depicts a seated man receiving a vigorous foot rub. Hippocrates, the Greek physician known as the father of modern medicine, was a fourth century B.C. proselytizer for massage. "The physician must be experienced in many things, but most assuredly in rubbing," he wrote.

BENEFITS EXPERIENCED BY:

The Giver: Giving a friend or loved one a foot massage is very soothing and calming for you, too, and can actually cause your blood pressure to decrease. It's a very caring, nurturing, and bonding experience to share with another person.

The Receiver: Obviously, this is really the best position to be in. Foot massage will help reduce your stress, boost circulation, and relieve blood stagnation from wearing ill-fitting shoes. In addition, it will dramatically relax your body, soothe foot muscles, undo knots and tension in your toes, balls of your feet, arches, and ankles, and soften your feet if a massage cream or oil is applied.

The Self-Massager: Though not as fulfilling as having your feet massaged by another, self-massage enables you to care for yourself on a regular basis, to de-stress, and to pamper your feet as you see fit.

BENEFITS OF FOOT MASSAGE

Regardless of whether you're on the receiving end of a foot massage or you're the one giving it, you both will experience many benefits. Even if you are simply massaging your own feet, it can still be a rewarding and satisfying way to end your day.

TECHNIQUES OF FOOT MASSAGE

A foot massage can be performed at any time you wish or as a part of your home pedicure procedure (see steps in chapter 8, page 161). The following illustrations depict some standard foot massage techniques that a nail technician might perform on her client during a pedicure. If you do not have a willing partner to give you a massage, never fear. These techniques are just as easily done (with a minor bit of alteration) by yourself on your own feet.

If a partner is involved, have the one receiving the foot massage recline against a big pillow on the sofa or bed to fully relax the entire body. Foot massage feels really great if the whole body is at ease.

If you're going solo, find a comfortable chair, preferably one with padded arms and a foot rest, such as a recliner. Sit back, prop one foot in your lap and let the other rest extended in front of you, and massage those feet until they smile or else you fall asleep!

Note: If using massage oil or lotion, a towel or two will come in handy to protect furniture and clothing.

Rub oiled or creamed hands together vigorously to warm them before beginning foot massage. Complete all six steps on one foot before moving on to the other.

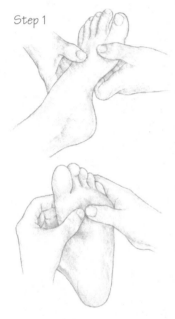

Step 1

Step 1: Stroking

Stimulates circulation and warms the foot. Holding your partner's foot in your hands, on the top of the foot begin a long, slow, firm stroking motion with your thumbs, starting at the tips of the toes and sliding back away from you, all the way to the ankle; then retrace your steps back to the toes with a lighter stroke. Repeat this step three to five times.

Now stroke the bottom of the foot with your thumbs, starting at the base of the toes and moving from the ball of the foot, over the arch, to the heel and then back again. Use long, firm strokes, slightly pressing the sole with your thumbs as you stroke. Repeat this step three to five times.

Step 2: Ankle Rotations

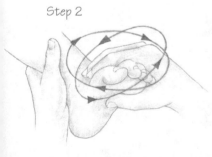

Step 2

Loosens joints and relaxes feet. Cup one hand under the heel, behind the ankle, to brace the foot and leg. Grasp the ball of the foot with the other hand and turn the foot slowly at the ankle for three to five times in each direction. With repeated foot massages, any stiffness will begin to recede. This is a particularly good exercise for those of you suffering from arthritis.

Step 3: Toe Pulls and Squeezes

Toes, like fingers, are quite sensitive to the touch. I find this massage step unbelievably calming. Grasp the foot beneath the arch. With the other hand, beginning with the big toe, hold the toe with your thumb on top and index finger beneath. Starting at the base of the toe, slowly and firmly pull the toe, sliding your fingers to the top and back to the base. Now repeat, but gently squeeze and roll the toe between your thumb and index finger, working your way to the tip and back to the base. Repeat these two movements on the remaining toes.

Step 4: Toe Slides

Grasp foot behind the ankle, cupping under heel. With the index finger of the other hand, insert your finger between toes, back and forth for three to five times.

Step 5: Arch Press

Releases tension in the inner and outer longitudinal arches. Hold foot as you did in step 4. Using heel of your other hand, push hard as you slide along the arch from the ball of the foot toward the heel and back again. Repeat five times. This part of the foot can stand a little extra exertion on your part, just don't apply too much pressure.

Step 6: Stroking

Repeat Step #1 above. This step is a good way to begin and end a foot massage.

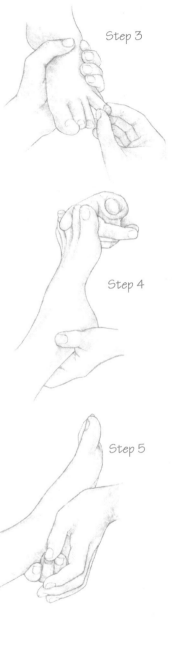

Step 3

Step 4

Step 5

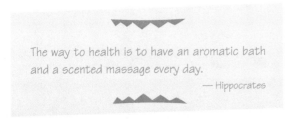

The way to health is to have an aromatic bath and a scented massage every day.

— Hippocrates

FOOT MASSAGE ELIXIR RECIPES

Foot massage can be performed with or without oils and creams. It's easier to grip your own or your partner's foot if it's dry, but I prefer to use a small amount of oil or cream fragranced with the essential oils I feel I need at that moment, and massage it in well, because my feet tend to be on the dry side. Don't overdo it, though, or the foot you are working on will be too slippery and difficult to hold.

The following recipes are very easy to make and have a relatively long shelf life in case you decide to double or triple the formula and store it for later use. The ingredients are especially good for dry, neglected feet and will leave your paws exceptionally soft and pampered. Enjoy!

POST-WORKOUT FOOT MASSAGE OIL

This formula will help feet feel cool and refreshed and aid in deodorizing.

2 teaspoons (10 ml) castor, soybean, jojoba, or extra-virgin olive oil

1 drop peppermint essential oil

1 drop eucalyptus essential oil

1 drop rosemary essential oil

Yield: 1 treatment

To make: Combine all ingredients in a small bowl. Stir thoroughly.

To use:

1. Use approximately 1 teaspoon (5 ml) per foot and massage in completely.

2. Put on socks after massage to absorb excess oil and soften feet.

DE-STRESSING FOOT BATH

Begin your mini–reflexology session with a soothing, sensory, and muscle-easing herbal foot bath to cleanse and soften your feet and take the edge off your nerves. I particularly like this one.

Foot tub
German chamomile
  flowers
Enough water to fill foot
  tub to ankle level
1/4 cup (60 ml) Epsom
  salts
1/4 cup (60 ml) baking
  soda
1 tablespoon (15 ml)
  borax
3–5 drops lavender,
  German chamomile,
  geranium, or clary sage

Yield: 1 treatment

To make:
1. Use ½ cup (120 ml) of dried German chamomile flowers for each gallon of water. Boil the water, remove from heat, and add German chamomile flowers. Cover and steep 5 to 10 minutes. Strain and cool until comfortable.
2. Pour all ingredients into foot tub and swish with feet to dissolve salts.
To use: Soak feet for at least 10 minutes. Pat dry. Reflexology is best practiced on dry feet.

Nothing can cure the soul but the senses, just as nothing can cure the senses but the soul.

—Oscar Wilde

CHAPTER 11
Common Foot Problems, Uncommon Remedies

$\blacktriangledown\blacktriangledown\blacktriangledown$

The American Podiatric Medical Association states, "Foot ailments are among the most common of our health problems. Although some can be traced to heredity, many stem from the cumulative impact of a lifetime of abuse and neglect. Studies show that 75 percent of Americans experience foot problems of a greater or lesser degree of seriousness at some time in their lives; nowhere near that many seek medical treatment, apparently because they mistakenly believe that discomfort and pain are normal and expectable."

Happy feet are healthy feet! Locate your foot problem(s) in the following pages and try the recommended natural remedies to help put your feet back on the path to comfort and wellness. If your tootsies need professional care, then follow the suggested foot specialist's advice and visit a podiatrist or orthopaedist if necessary.

To find further foot health information, contact The American Podiatric Medical Association, The American Academy of Podiatric Sports Medicine, or The American Orthopaedic Foot and Ankle Society and ask for their informative foot health brochures. I found them all to be very professional and quite helpful while doing research on the foot.

You might also want to look in the Yellow Pages under "Physicians (M.D.)" for an orthopaedic surgeon/orthopaedist, or "Physicians (D.P.M.)" for a podiatrist.

- Avoid a highly stressful lifestyle. Stress can sometimes aggravate an existing arthritic condition.
- Avoid smoking, excess caffeine, soda, alcohol, protein, and fat.
- Most importantly, keep your doctor informed of any changes in the condition of your feet.

SOOTHING HERBAL POULTICE

This wonderful herbal recipe helps to relieve the pain and inflammation of swollen joints in the feet. It revs up the circulation and helps ease stiffness and pain. I based it on several formulas I discovered that were used over a century ago. All herbs called for are in dry form.

2 tablespoons (30 ml) plantain leaves

3 tablespoons (45 ml) powdered marsh mallow root

1 tablespoon (15 ml) powdered meadowsweet leaves

1 teaspoon (5 ml) powdered cayenne pepper

Yield: 1 treatment

To make:

1. Combine all ingredients in a medium-sized bowl.

2. Add enough boiling water to form a paste. Stir until you have a gooey consistency and paste feels slippery. Allow to cool a bit if too hot to comfortably touch.

To use:

1. Spread paste on a piece of flannel and place over the swollen joint(s). Wrap the area with plastic wrap. Cover with a warm towel that's right out of the dryer or microwave, if possible. Sit in a comfortable chair, elevate your foot, and relax for about 30 minutes or longer.

2. When finished, rinse your foot and apply a good thick cream to both feet and ankles. Then put on socks.

FOOT FACT

According to the American Orthopaedic Foot and Ankle Society, almost half of people in their sixties and seventies have arthritis of the foot and/or ankle.

See a Physician If: If you notice joint stiffness, tenderness, or swelling in your normally healthy feet, visit your foot specialist for a diagnosis. Early diagnosis and treatment may help prevent the situation from developing further.

If your minor arthritis takes a turn for the worse and walking becomes increasingly painful and joints become red or inflamed, by all means schedule an appointment immediately.

Your physician can work with you to design a treatment plan to help preserve joint function or possibly restore it if it's been lost, and help control pain and inflammation. You may want to seek out a holistic foot specialist who uses nutritional and herbal therapies in conjunction with allopathic medicine to help heal your condition.

ATHLETE'S FOOT

Athlete's foot is so named because this infection was most commonly seen on the feet of athletes who spent time around swimming pools, steam baths, locker rooms, and showers following exercise. These places are a breeding ground for fungus, and so are your shoes because the environment inside is dark, warm, and moist. Athlete's foot has become more commonplace since the 1970s due to increased interest in fitness and exercise.

Causes: *Tinea pedis*, the Latin name for fungal foot infection, is a skin disease caused by dermatophytes (tiny parasitic fungi) that thrive in warm, moist places. It usually occurs between the toes and on the soles of the feet.

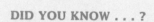

DID YOU KNOW . . . ?

Athlete's foot affects approximately nineteen million adults per year, mostly male.

Symptoms: The symptoms can appear rather quickly and can include scaling, flaking, and peeling of the skin between the toes, intense itching, heat, redness, cracking, dryness, and finally the appearance of blisters if the disease is allowed to progress without treatment. The blisters can break and allow the fungus to enter below the skin's surface, thus making the disease even more difficult to treat. Athlete's foot symptoms tend to recur quite easily once you've been infected.

Treatment: A cure for this miserable skin affliction can sometimes be quite elusive because the pesky fungi can penetrate beneath the skin's surface and be difficult to reach with topical treatments. Because they don't penetrate deeply enough to reach the bloodstream, oral medications can have a tough time too. All treatments for athlete's foot should be taken or applied continuously over a period of several weeks to several months until the condition remedies itself.

A simple herbal remedy to try consists of 2 teaspoons (10 ml) tincture of benzoin combined with a few drops of lavender and thyme essential oils, which can help to heal any open cracks on your feet and kill the fungus. Massage this mixture in thoroughly between your toes and on the soles of your feet and allow to dry. Follow this treatment with a good foot cream.

HAPPY FEET

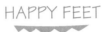

Try this recipe, contributed by an herbalist friend of mine, Jean Argus, to fight foot fungus and odor. It's terrific for active folks!

1 cup (250 ml) cornstarch
2 cups (500 ml) bentonite clay
2 tablespoons (30 ml) powdered goldenseal root
3 tablespoons (45 ml) powdered chaparral leaves
2 tablespoons (30 ml) powdered myrrh gum
4 tablespoons (60 ml) powdered black walnut hulls
3 tablespoons (45 ml) powdered thyme leaves
1 teaspoon (5 ml) peppermint essential oil

Yield: approximately 4 cups (1 liter)

To make:
Mix all ingredients and add essential oil a few drops at a time, blending well.

To use:
Sprinkle this healthful formula daily onto feet and into shoes.

Storage:
Store in a shaker container and use within one year for maximum potency.

Garlic is a potent antifungal and antibiotic and can be used internally and externally in the war against these fungi. Garlic oil can be very effective against athlete's foot and can be purchased in capsule form from the health food store. Simply pierce the capsules and rub the oil onto your affected feet. The oil can also be made fresh at home with this recipe.

ANTIFUNGAL GARLIC OIL

1 cup (250 ml) extra-virgin olive oil

20 peeled and pressed garlic cloves

30 drops tea tree essential oil

15 drops clove essential oil

30 drops lavender essential oil

Yield: approximately 1 cup (250 ml)

To make:

1. Place the olive oil and pressed garlic mash into a small pan over low heat; cover. Allow the garlic to infuse for 1 to 2 hours. The oil should get hot, just shy of a simmer. By then your kitchen will smell pleasantly pungent!

2. Remove from the heat and allow to cool. Strain, add essential oils, and stir. Keep refrigerated in a tightly capped bottle for up to 6 weeks.

To use: You could massage a tablespoon (15 ml) into your feet each morning, put on your socks and go off to work, but the stench would follow you around all day. Instead I recommend applying the oil at night after you've thoroughly washed and dried your feet; then slip on a pair of clean socks and go to bed. I can almost guarantee you won't have any romantic encounters while undergoing this treatment! As the garlic penetrates your feet, it will begin to show up on your breath. This treatment should be performed nightly for approximately 2 to 4 weeks.

Orally, garlic capsules can be taken to boost your immune system and fight the battle from the inside. Allicin, one of garlic's important chemicals, is responsible for its antifungal action. The recommended dosage is four to eight capsules, preferably spread throughout the day, taken with a large quantity of water. Garlic has a tendency to upset sensitive stomachs and cause gas, so you be the judge as to what your tolerance level is. It can't hurt you. The only problem with garlic is that you inherit the lovely fumes along with the benefits.

Prevention: Here are several tips to help you avoid contracting this infection:

- Wear shower shoes or rubber thongs when using public showers, walking in locker rooms and around public swimming pools, or lounging around in the steam room. Fungi thrive in these warm, damp, humid places.
- Wash and dry your feet daily.
- Change socks and shoes during the day if you perspire heavily.
- If overweight, lose it. Overweight people tend to sweat profusely, and are more prone to athlete's foot than people of normal weight.
- If diabetic, be especially watchful for athlete's foot. The sugar in your perspiration is the perfect feeding ground for fungus to proliferate.
- Athlete's foot is contagious to other people as well as to other body parts of your own. To avoid spreading this fungus among us, either dry your feet with paper towels and throw them away or immediately launder your foot-only drying towel in hot water. Bath mats should not be kept in the bathroom if you share this room with other family members. Use clean towels as temporary bath mats and also launder them immediately.
- Wear open-toed shoes as often as possible. Feet can breathe and stay drier this way.
- Sprinkle a little powder in your shoes daily to keep your feet fresh and dry.

See a Physician If: Several other skin problems can masquerade themselves as athlete's foot, such as a skin allergy or problems resulting from diabetes, circulatory disorders, drug abuse, stress, or poor nutrition. If these have been ruled out and self-treatment is not curing the disease, see a foot specialist or dermatologist immediately. They can prescribe topical or oral antifungal drugs to use in conjunction with all of the above treatments and preventative measures. As with any drug, especially antifungal drugs, there are side effects, which include liver toxicity.

BLACK TOENAILS

Causes: Black toenails (subungual hematoma) are caused by an injury to the toenail. Stubbing the toe against a hard object or dropping something heavy on it can cause a black toenail to form. Athletes, especially runners, frequently experience this malady. This toenail injury can occur if their shoes are too short or by running downhill, thus forcing the toes to repeatedly jam up against the inside of the shoe.

Symptoms: As blood pools under the injured nail (this is what causes the black color) and pressure builds, this sometimes results in pain. Most times, black toenails are not painful, just unsightly.

Treatment: Foot specialists recommend a procedure that you can perform at home to release the pooled blood and relieve the pressure under the toenail. Just thinking about this treatment leaves me feeling a bit woozy, but I will mention it here.

The toenail can usually be saved if the blood is drained. First, clean your foot thoroughly, dry, and swab the affected toe with alcohol. Next, heat the end of a needle or a paper clip with a match until it is red hot. If you're brave, now gently pierce your toenail. The heat from the sharp object melts the nail and allows the blood to flow out from beneath it. Follow this procedure with a hot foot bath and add a few drops of lavender or tea tree essential oil as a disinfectant. Dry your feet and swab the toe with alcohol or tincture of benzoin and a drop of tea tree essential oil. If your toenail *does* begin to loosen over time, cushion the nail with gauze and tape it down with an adhesive bandage (don't stick tape to the toenail itself or you may rip the nail off when you remove the bandage). This prevents your toenail from catching on your hosiery or socks.

Caution: Never perform this type of self-treatment if you have circulatory problems or are diabetic. See your physician immediately.

Prevention: The best way to prevent a black toenail is to be more graceful and not drop things on your toes or run into things . . . and also to buy proper fitting shoes. Your shoes should have a roomy toe box that allows your toes to wiggle and has about a half inch of space between your toes and the end of the shoe.

See a Physician If: If you can't possibly envision yourself piercing your toenail with a hot object, or if swelling and infection set in, then see a doctor.

SEASONAL FOOT LESION?

Walter J. Pedowitz, M.D., has found that in his practice, the incidence of black toenails increases dramatically around Thanksgiving and Easter! These are the two holidays when people remove 12- to 18-pound (5- to 8-kilogram) frozen turkeys from the freezer, and drop them square on their big toe! OUCH!

BLISTERS

Causes: Everyone has had a blister at one time or another. They are caused by friction against the skin from a shoe, abrasive socks, or hosiery and can develop on any part of the foot, even the tips of your toes. New leather shoes are notorious for causing blisters because they tend to be snug until the leather stretches a bit, but any type of footwear can cause a blister, whether the shoe is too big, too short, or too narrow. Runners, walkers, and rollerbladers tend to get more blisters than sedentary folk. All that foot movement and pounding can cause the feet to swell and sweat inside the shoe, resulting in lots of blister-causing friction.

Symptoms: You can actually feel when a blister is beginning to form. The spot gets warm, then irritated, then downright painful if you don't remove your shoe. These whitish pockets of skin filled with clear fluid form between the skin's inner and outer layers in response to friction and can make walking unbearable.

Treatment: There seem to be different schools of thought on whether to pop a blister or not. Some say to leave it alone, whether large or small. Wash the area and swab it with alcohol or iodine; then cover it with an adhesive bandage or moleskin, remove the source of friction, and let nature take her course. Other physicians and sports injury specialists suggest that by popping the blister, especially a large one, healing will take place faster. If a blister breaks on its own, treat the same as if you'd just popped it (see below).

To open a blister, first wash and dry your foot thoroughly. Swab the blister with alcohol or other disinfectant and carefully puncture the edge with a flame-sterilized needle or razor blade. Now drain the fluid, but don't peel off any skin. Allow the layers of skin to adhere. Cleanse with disinfectant again and dry. Apply a bandage, but remove it at night to allow the blister to breathe and dry out, and reapply in the morning after your shower. If it stays moist, healing is postponed and infection can set in.

Caution: Don't attempt self-treatment if you have circulatory problems or are diabetic.

Prevention: Irritating blisters are easy to prevent. Here are some tips for avoiding them:

- Buy well-fitting shoes. Ideally they should not rub anywhere, even from the beginning. Add insoles or heel cushions if necessary.
- If you are blister prone or performing lots of physical activity, always wear good socks and apply adhesive felt or moleskin to areas on your feet that frequently blister.
- Sprinkle powder into shoes and/or socks daily to reduce friction.
- Some people swear by petroleum jelly or vegetable shortening as a blister preventative. Try the Blister Resister Cream recipe on page 187.

See a Physician If: Blisters are rarely serious. If the blister develops inflammation or an infection, see your doctor immediately.

BLISTER RESISTER CREAM

⅓ cup (80 ml) all-
  vegetable shortening
10 drops eucalyptus
  essential oil
10 drops camphor essen-
  tial oil
Optional: If you're a peppermint lover, like me,
  you can substitute 15
  to 20 drops of pep-
  permint essential oil
  instead of the above-
  listed oils.

Yield: about ⅓ cup (80 ml)

To make: Beat ingredients together with a spoon or small whisk.

To use: Apply to blister-prone areas, then cover with thick socks. Helps reduce friction between the sensitive spot and your shoe.

Storage: Store in a small glass or plastic jar and label. Keep refrigerated if not used within thirty days.

BLISTER BUSTIN' FOOT POWDER

This herbal foot powder is simple to make.

½ cup (125 ml) white clay
½ cup (125 ml) corn-
  starch
1 tablespoon (15 ml)
  finely powdered sage
  leaves
1 tablespoon (15 ml)
  finely powdered pep-
  permint leaves
½ teaspoon (2 ml) clove
  or peppermint essen-
  tial oil

Yield: slightly more than
1 cup (250 ml)

To make:

1. In a medium-sized bowl, whisk togeth-er the clay, cornstarch, sage, and pepper-mint. You can also use a food processor set on the lowest setting if you wish.

2. Add the essential oil a few drops at a time and thoroughly blend.

To use: Sprinkle this spicy powder into your shoes each morning or into your socks to help keep friction, moisture, and odor to a minimum.

Storage: Store in a shaker container and use within one year.

BUNION OF THE BIG TOE

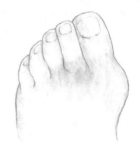

Causes: There is no single cause of a bunion. It may develop from arthritic joint destruction, overpronation of the foot, heredity, or from wearing ill-fitting, tight shoes.

Symptoms: A bunion (or *hallux valgus*) is an inflammation and thickening of the bursa of the joint of the big toe, frequently associated with enlargement of the joint and deformity of the toe. It results in ugly, misshapen feet with the big toe angling in and either tucking under or over your second toe. It is usually painless but can be quite painful if allowed to progress. A bunion has the tendency to increase in size due to excessive weight load and from shoe pressure. It causes widening of the forefoot and may cause your gait to become off-balance. Though not as commonplace, a bunion on your small toe is called a tailor's bunion.

Treatment: Sometimes merely changing the type of shoes you wear can prevent the worsening of a bunion. Whether you are a man or woman, switching from a tight, pointed toe shoe to a sandal can help tremendously. So can wearing a *bunion shoe,* available from most orthopedic shoe stores. Both shoe styles remove the source of pressure on the bunion and have a wider forefront to accommodate a bunioned foot. If you refuse to change shoe styles due to vanity, then your bunion will progressively get bigger, uglier, and eventually painful.

If athletic, you can make a slit in the shoe in the bunion area to allow for extra room and less pressure. If necessary, try a commercial arch support to help take some of the weight off the bunion.

Try placing a pad over the bunion to reduce friction. You don't want to add thickness though, as this would just add more pressure, so cut a hole in the middle of the pad where the bunion protrudes. The surrounding area is now built up a bit and hopefully some pressure is taken off the bunion.

Prevention: If bunions run in your family, you can dramatically slow the progression by wearing well-fitting, non-binding, low-heeled shoes with a wide toebox. In fact, everyone should heed this advice. Most of today's fashionable shoes are designed for an elf's foot — long and pointy — not a human's foot. Shoe designers should be ashamed for trying to force your foot into a shape it was never meant to be in and for trying to dictate fashion styles. You should be allowed the freedom to wear comfortable shoes with your work clothes without inciting derision from co-workers and a reprimand from the personnel director.

See a Physician If: If you've tried self-treatment and your bunion is still getting worse and possibly painful, see your foot specialist. He or she may want to rule out osteoarthritis, rheumatoid arthritis, gout, or infection first, as these can also cause pain and inflammation in the big toe. Foot surgery may be required if your bunion is disabling and your foot severely disfigured.

CALLUSES

Causes: Calluses can be caused by wearing shoes that are too tight, too short, or even too big and sloppy. They can even be caused by going barefoot a lot. Anything that causes rubbing, pressure, or pinching of the skin on your foot can result in a callus. Approximately 14 percent of adults get calluses annually; it's a very common malady.

Symptoms: Calluses are thickened, raised layers of hard, tough, yellow-reddish brown dead skin, oval or elongated in shape, that form on the bottom of your foot, heel, side of your big toe, or even the tips of your toes as a defense mechanism against repeated friction and pressure from rubbing against your shoes or seams in your socks. They can become painful if allowed to grow very thick.

Treatment: The only way to permanently remove a callus is to remove the cause. So unless you're totally sedentary and bedridden, you will more than likely have a callus or two or three on your feet. Calluses return and return, no matter how often you scrape them off. They keep pedicurists in business.

Personally, I use a foot file with medium grit sand paper on one side and fine grit on the other to file down the dead skin on my heels and balls of my feet three times a week. I do this while standing in the shower after the skin has softened a bit. This procedure could also be performed while sitting on the edge of the tub after soaking your feet for a few minutes in ankle-high water. If you add a cup (250 ml) of baking soda or vinegar to the tub, your feet will be even softer. I then dry my feet with a rough toweling and follow with thick moisturizer. I'm very callus prone and this practice keeps my tootsies relatively soft and pain free. A pumice stone can be used in place of the foot file, though I find my file much easier to handle.

Better drug stores carry a tool called a corn and callus trimmer, which is specially made for removing thick calluses. It holds a razor blade or a series of small blades and is used by gently scraping the blade(s) over the softened, callused skin. Extreme caution should be taken when using this tool so that you do not cut too deeply and draw blood.

Moleskin and adhesive felt can be custom cut and placed around the callus to help take the pressure off and relieve the pain and irritation.

Caution: Diabetics, people with circulatory problems, and those with unsteady hands should never attempt to cut or scrape their calluses.

An herbalist friend of mine, Julie Bailey, owner of Mountain Rose Herbs (see Resources), kindly let me borrow her enchanting, mystical recipe for making calendula oil. Try to make 4 to 5 cups (1 to 1.25 liters) of this super healing oil so you can have plenty for other formulas throughout this book. She also sells this wonderful oil ready-made if you're short on time!

"Three days before the moon is full, gather the golden flowers (calendula) after the dew dries but before the noonday sun. Thank the energies, spirits or devas; whom or whichever calls to you. Spread the golden flowers on a screen in a dry, shady and well-ventilated place to wilt and lose most of their water. (They should be leathery, not crisp.)

"On the evening of the full moon, select a thoroughly clean glass jar that will be two thirds full with the golden flowers. Choose the best cold-pressed, extra-virgin olive oil. Pour the oil over the flowers to almost three thirds. Put the lid on tight. Dance and sing to the oil. Shake the oil.

"Place your oil in a sun box (greenhouse, hot water closet, black sand pit, etc.). Visit your oil every few days. Dance, sing, and shake. One day before the next full moon, bring your oil into the kitchen. Strain your oil. Bottle every drop into clean dark glass bottles and label.

"Congratulations! You have created and participated in medicine and magic."

This is actually my preferred method of making my herbal oils. It may not be scientific, but I feel that by allowing the universal energy systems to create my healing potion according to their timetable, not mine, I receive a super-charged medicine, a true gift from Mother Earth herself! She provides the medicinal plants and the solar energy. I simply join them together and reap the benefits!

Note: Some water from the herb may still be left in the oil. If, after 2 weeks, you see what looks like dirt in the bottom of the jar of strained oil, that's water settling. This can make your oil go rancid. Pour the oil into a fresh jar, stopping before the "dirt" pours in. Repeat this process a few times until the oil stays clear.

Prevention: There are really only four simple rules to follow to help prevent calluses from forming:

- Take good care of your feet. Inspect them daily for developing calluses and other foot problems, and treat accordingly.
- Wear shoes that fit.
- Don't walk barefoot on hard surfaces such as asphalt or concrete for any length of time or protective calluses will form on the soles of your feet.
- If overweight, lose it. The combination of excess weight and ill-fitting shoes puts way too much pressure on your poor feet and encourages callus formation.

See a Physician If: If your calluses are not responding to home treatment and keep worsening and become painful, see a foot specialist. Diabetic and elderly people frequently need assistance with foot care because of circulatory problems or because they just can't bend over to scrub the rough spots. Also, the callus(es) may not be just the result of friction, but could be forming because of a foot misalignment problem, which would need to be treated.

CALENDULA BLOSSOM OIL

An alternate, quicker method for making herbal oils is to use the stove method. Here's what you need:

4–5 cups (1 to 1.25 liters) calendula blossoms (wilted in well-ventilated shade for 24 hours)
Extra-virgin olive oil

Yield: About 4 cups (1 liter)

To make:

1. Put the calendula blossoms in a 3-quart (3 liter) pot and pour in enough olive oil to cover by 2 inches (5 cm). The mixture should look almost like a flower-head paste, but with enough oil to allow the flowers to move about slightly.

2. Turn the burner on low. Heat the mixture just below a simmer, and allow to steep for 5 to 10 hours. Don't put a lid on the pot. This only traps in any moisture left in the flowers and will introduce it into your herbal oil, which will encourage spoilage. Check on it every hour or so to make sure the oil isn't simmering.

3. Remove from the heat after the oil smells herby and has attained a rich, golden-orange color.

4. Cool, strain, bottle, label, and refrigerate.

To use: You now have a potent healing oil that can be used as a base in any recipe calling for oil in this section of the book. Try some in the next recipe.

Storage: Will keep 6 months to 1 year if refrigerated. Use within 60 days if not refrigerated.

CALLUS SMOOTHER SCRUB

1 tablespoon (15 ml) sea
  salt
1 tablespoon (15 ml)
  calendula oil
5 drops orange or
  spearmint essential oil

Yield: 1 treatment

To make: In a small bowl, combine all ingredients until the salt is completely covered by the oil.

To use:

1. First, soak and wash your feet in order to soften the dead, callused skin. Pat dry.

2. While sitting on the edge of the tub or over a towel or foot tub, massage the mixture into your feet, scrubbing with a moderately firm hand over your callused areas. Do this for as long as you want, but at least 2 to 3 minutes per foot.

3. Rinse with warm water and roughly rub your feet dry. You should now have a moisturizing calendula oil residue remaining on your feet that will penetrate and continue to soften for hours to come.

4. Massage a bit of castor oil into each foot and put on a pair of socks if you want to really pamper your feet.

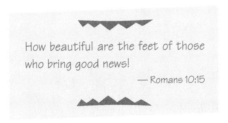

How beautiful are the feet of those who bring good news!

— Romans 10:15

CHILDREN'S FOOT PROBLEMS

Many adult foot ailments begin in childhood. This is why it is paramount that you see to it that your child's feet are properly cared for. Neglecting foot health when young can lead to leg and back problems later in life. Children's feet grow very rapidly. By 12 to 16 months, their feet have reached almost half adult size. This is a critical time to really pay attention to foot health and head off any potential development problems.

Children can suffer from some of the same foot problems as adults, including athlete's foot, profuse perspiration and odor, sports injuries, and wounds or scrapes from running around barefoot.

Causes, Symptoms, and Treatment: The causes, symptoms, and treatment of most foot problems are the same in children as adults. However, because the bones in children's feet are not completely hardened, sports injuries can be especially damaging. Their feet are soft and pliable, and excess pressure from playing the same sport over and over or from training too long and hard can cause long-term problems. Your child could become injury prone. Many doctors recommend that the intense, specialized sports training be postponed until the late teens, after growth plates are closed.

If perspiration and odor are a problem, make sure to have your child wash his or her feet two to three times a day, wear clean cotton or wool socks, and sprinkle powder into shoes and socks every day.

Prevention: Most importantly, make sure your children take a daily bath and thoroughly clean their feet. Check for tenderness, minor irritations, calluses or corns developing (which could be a sign that they are outgrowing their shoes), or rashes (a possible sign of poison ivy or athlete's foot). Trim long toenails. Check to see how their shoes fit. Is there enough room in the toe box for their toes to wiggle? If not, invest in a new pair. And, give them a gentle foot massage once a

FOOT FACT

Have you ever looked at a newborn's feet? They're small and pudgy and relatively flat. All toddlers under 16 months have flat feet. Their arches don't fully develop until they reach seven or eight years of age.

week if they're receptive. It'll let you take a good look at the condition of their feet, and it's good bonding time to boot!

See a Physician If: If you notice something that looks abnormal in your child's feet, see a foot specialist. Poor posture, an awkward or stumbling gait, toes that turn in or out, knock knees, or bowleggedness can be a sign that something is amiss. Many times a child will outgrow these problems, but it's better to be safe than sorry. Serious deformities such as clubfoot or skew foot should be treated as soon as possible.

FUNGUS AMONG US OIL

Here's a nighttime herbal treatment to help clear up athlete's foot in children.

2 teaspoons (10 ml) castor, jojoba, soybean, or extra-virgin olive oil

2 drops tea tree essential oil

1 drop lavender essential oil

1 drop clove or thyme essential oil

Yield: 1 treatment

To make: Stir oils together in a small bowl.

To use:

1. Thoroughly massage the oil into your child's clean feet (the child can do it if older). Concentrate between toes and around cuticles. If only one foot is infected, treat the other one anyway as a preventative.

2. Put on socks and send the little one off to bed. Do this nightly for several weeks until healing takes place.

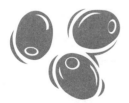

DR. MOM'S HERBAL HEALING CREAM

For minor scrapes, scratches, bug bites, and small puncture wounds from running through the woods and stepping on thorns and pinecones, keep this healing cream on hand. It's extremely soothing and moisturizing for your child's playtime injuries as well as excellent for your dry hands, elbows, knees, legs, and feet. It's also the best cuticle conditioner I've ever made!

½ cup (125 ml) distilled water
2 teaspoons (10 ml) chopped comfrey root
2 teaspoons (10 ml) plantain leaves
¾ teaspoon (4 ml) borax
½ cup (125 ml) vegetable shortening
1 teaspoon (5 ml) beeswax
15 drops lavender or geranium essential oil
5 drops orange essential oil

Yield: approximately ¾ cup (180 ml)

Note: If using fresh herbs, decrease the water by 2 tablespoons and double the herb portions.

To make:

1. Add water and herbs to a small saucepan, cover, and simmer on a very low setting for 30 minutes.

2. Add the borax and stir until dissolved. Remove from heat and cool until just warm.

3. While the herbs are cooling, melt the vegetable shortening and beeswax in another small saucepan over low heat until just melted. Do not allow to simmer.

4. Remove from heat and stir in essential oils.

5. Strain the herbs through a mesh strainer lined with pantyhose or cheesecloth, reserving the greenish herbal liquid in a cup. Gently lift the liner material and twist and squeeze the healing, slippery mucilage out into the container. You should have approximately ¼ to ⅓ cup (60 to 80 ml) of herbal formula. Dispose of the herbs into your garden or atop a house plant.

6. By now the herbal liquid and melted vegetable shortening should be approximately the same temperature. While briskly stirring the shortening with one

hand, slowly drizzle in the herbal liquid with the other. Continue stirring until creamy and almost firm. If you set your small saucepan over a bowl of ice while performing this procedure, it will set up quite quickly. You should now have an approximate ¾ cup (180 ml) of multipurpose cream. It will have a pale greenish-brown color and smell pleasantly herby.

To use: Apply this cream generously over cleaned, irritated skin. Use as often as you wish. My skin drinks it right up. It doesn't tend to be greasy, unless too much is used.

Storage: Store in decorative glass or plastic jars and refrigerate. Discard if not used within 45 days.

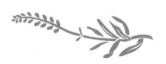

COLD FEET

It seems that women tend to suffer more from cold feet than men. Is it because women frequently wear tight shoes that restrict circulation to the feet? It may be that women in their menstruating years can suffer from iron deficiency, which results in a lower level of oxygen-carrying red blood cells traveling throughout the muscle tissue, impairing circulation to the feet. Whatever the cause, having cold feet can be downright uncomfortable. I've elicited agonizing screams from my husband when I've placed my winter-frigid feet on his toasty back in bed. He hates it, but it feels so good to me!

Causes: Cold feet can also be a result of pneumonia, heart failure, diabetes, malnutrition, injury, or nervous system impairment.

Symptoms: I don't have to tell you how cold feet feel . . . COLD! They are also chilly to the touch, sometimes tingly and a bit numb, and can even be a bit bluish or purple in color due to poor circulation.

Treatment: Walk, walk, walk! Keep those feet moving and your heart pumping as often and for as many miles as possible. The more you move, the better your circulation. That's the key to having warm feet.

Make sure you include plenty of foods containing vitamins A, B complex, C, D, E, and iron, in your daily diet. These nutrients, in particular, strengthen the veins and capillaries and help keep your blood oxygen-rich.

Another remedy that you may have heard of is to sprinkle powdered cayenne pepper into your shoes and socks. This is a stimulating, warming herb and will cause increased circulation to the feet. Mix about 2 teaspoons (10 ml) white cosmetic clay, cornstarch, or arrowroot with 1 teaspoon (5 ml) powdered cayenne pepper and sprinkle away. Be sure to wash your hands thoroughly after handling cayenne. Also, acquire a taste for hot sauce or hot peppers such as jalapeño or habañero. By simply adding these tasty foods to your diet, you will automatically rev up your circulation and add lots of vitamins C and A as well.

Prevention: Here are a few tips to ensure nice warm tootsies:

♦ Always wear comfortable shoes, never too tight or too short.
♦ Keep feet warm and dry by wearing socks that breathe; natural fibers are best.
♦ Get plenty of exercise and fresh air and breathe deeply.
♦ Eat a nutritious, well-balanced diet.
♦ If you sit or stand in one position all day long, get up and stretch your feet and legs periodically to keep the blood from stagnating in your legs.

See a Physician If: If you suddenly start suffering from cold feet or are a chronic sufferer and none of the above suggestions seem to help, schedule a doctor's visit. Your doctor may want to rule out a circulatory disorder, anemia, or diabetes.

HOT AND COLD FOOT BATH THERAPY

Here's an invigorating, old-fashioned remedy for cold feet. It wakes up the entire body, too!

2 foot bath tubs
2 tablespoons (30 ml)
   peppermint leaves
2 tablespoons (30 ml)
   rosemary leaves
2 bath towels

Yield: 1 treatment

To make:

1. Bring to boil enough water to fill one foot tub. Remove from heat and add herbs tightly tied in cheesecloth. Cover and steep for 15 minutes. Remove the herb bags.

2. Find a comfortable chair and place a bath towel on the floor in front of it and put the foot tubs, side-by-side, on the towel. Fill one tub with the hot herbal liquid and the other with almost icy water. Throw in a few ice cubes if you wish, since you're going to be sitting here for a while.

To use:

1. Put feet in the hot tub first for 3 to 5 minutes (careful, don't scald yourself), then immerse in the cold water for 30 seconds or so. Alternate 2 to 3 times.

2. When finished, briskly rub feet dry with a coarse towel for about 1 minute per foot.

3. Slather on a rich moisturizer, and put on thick wool or cotton socks. Your feet should feel great.

Caution: If diabetic, please don't partake of this foot bath. Because of the temperature extremes, it can potentially cause a sugar imbalance and possible dizziness.

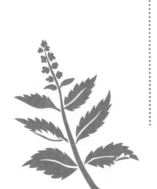

CORNS

Causes: If you could go barefoot every day of your life, you wouldn't get corns. Corns are caused by pressure or friction from ill-fitting shoes. But unless you live wild and free in a temperate climate, shoes are a required and necessary part of your dress code. Unlike a wart, a corn does not contain blood vessels or nerve endings. People with a cavus foot type or extremely high arch are often susceptible to this affliction because their toes are pulled back a bit and corns tend to form on the tips and tops of the toes as well.

Symptoms: A hard corn, or *heloma durum,* is a tough, cone-shaped thickening of the horny layer of the epidermis that usually occurs over a toe joint, having a hard, brownish-gray "eye" in the center and surrounded by inflamed skin.

A soft corn, or *heloma molle,* forms between the toes as a result of friction. It is soft because the sweat between your toes softens the normally hard corn tissue. Beneath every corn there is a prominence of the bone, so when your toes are squeezed together, such as when wearing narrow, tight flat shoes or pointed-toe, high-heeled shoes, the bones will rub against each other, causing pressure and irritation. As a result, layers of tissue grow over the pressure point(s) until a corn or two are formed. The constant friction between your toes causes the skin of the soft corn to die or become inflamed, which can lead to very painful walking.

Treatment: You can either change your shoe style and take the pressure off your corns so they'll go away on their own, or continue to perform constant maintenance on your existing and new corns.

Corn pads are available from the drugstore. These have a hole cut out of the middle so the padding fits around the corn and the pressure is relieved. Corn pads take up space, so make sure to wear roomier shoes while wearing the pad. Custom pads can also be

FOOT FACT

Your feet tend to widen and change shape as you age. They should be measured whenever new shoes are purchased to help avoid the development of blisters, bunions, corns, calluses, and other foot problems that can stem from shoes that are too tight or ill-fitting.

made from moleskin and adhesive felt, as thick or as thin as you wish, but always put the padding around the corn, not on top of it.

For women who feel they must wear high heels, some pressure can be relieved by placing a metatarsal pad in front of the heads of your metatarsals to prevent your toes from sliding down and jamming into the pointed-toe portion of your shoe. This will reduce *some* of the friction, but definitely not all of it.

Some foot specialists disagree as to whether to apply salicylic ointment or drops (also known as corn drops), available from the drugstore, to your corns. The drops *can* help remove the corn, but if any of the acid runs off onto the surrounding skin, it can burn and even cause a hole or ulcer to form. The drops can be applied in the center of the corn pad, but please use with care.

Caution: Diabetics should never use salicylic acid drops to treat corns. Ulceration of the skin could lead to serious problems.

In his book *American Folk Medicine* (Meyerbooks, Glenwood, Illinois, 1973), Clarence Meyer includes a corn remedy used by Dr. R. L. Louis in 1877: "Take bark of the common willow, burn to ashes, mix them with strong vinegar and apply to the parts. This is a very effectual remedy for corns or warts." The reason this might work is that acetic acid, the main constituent of vinegar, applied daily to the corn will soften the dead skin and cause the corn to slowly peel away. Straight vinegar can also be used. Try it and see if it works for you.

FOOT FACT

Every year approximately 150 million people get corns, though only a fraction seek professional treatment.

Other old-fashioned remedies include applying wintergreen essential oil to soft corns and wrapping soft linen around the toe or swabbing hard corns with castor oil and also wrapping with linen. Do these daily until the corns disappear.

Prevention: Stop wearing shoes that pinch or bind. Wear open-toed sandals or comfortable shoes with a wide toe box. Go barefoot as much as possible, either on the grass or beach or around the house, so your feet can expand and relax.

See a Physician If: If a corn reaches the painful stage and nothing seems to be helping, your foot specialist can extract it for you. Your doctor can also trim it, if you feel you can't do it yourself, though it is almost certain to return if you continue to wear the same shoe style. If the problem persists, your doctor may need to perform surgery.

DIABETIC FOOT CONCERNS

Causes and Symptoms: Diabetes is relatively unknown in poorer countries where food is scarce and overeating is not a problem, but in the United States, the land of plenty, it is one of the major degenerative diseases, afflicting approximately sixteen million people. It is a metabolic disease characterized by high blood sugar and the inability to properly process dietary carbohydrates, resulting in an abnormal amount of sugar in the urine. Health problems, such as cardiovascular disease, obesity, retinopathy, blindness, kidney damage, and circulatory disorders of the limbs and feet, often develop as the illness progresses.

Diabetics frequently suffer from foot problems such as athlete's foot, neuropathy, numbness, cold feet, ulceration, calluses, and corns. It is therefore wise to visit a foot specialist at least twice a year to prevent any minor problems from developing into potentially limb-threatening complications.

Diabetics, like everyone else, can have a problem with athlete's foot, but because the perspiration of the diabetic person is "sweet" from the increased sugar in the blood, it makes a doubly fun place for the fungus to frolic. See "Athlete's Foot" on page 180 for treatment suggestions.

Neuropathy is the gradual loss of nerve function in the legs and feet leading to loss of feeling or sensation. It can also affect the ankles and hands. If you have this disease, you won't be able to feel if you've injured your foot or if blisters have formed from snug shoes. Loss of feeling in the feet of a diabetic can lead to serious problems down the road.

Poor circulation of the lower limbs can slow the healing process. What might start as a minor cut, bruise, blister, corn, or callus could develop into an open sore, infection, ulceration, and eventually gangrene if not properly cared for. Diabetics frequently suffer from cold feet and hands. Your situation

VANILLA FOOT BUTTER

4 tablespoons (60 ml) almond, olive, jojoba, soybean, or calendula oil

1 vanilla bean, chopped into ¼ inch (.6 cm) pieces (available in grocery or health food stores)

1 tablespoon (15 ml) beeswax

2 tablespoons (30 ml) cocoa butter

1 tablespoon (15 ml) anhydrous lanolin

20 drops geranium, rosemary, or peppermint essential oil

Yield: approximately ½ cup (125 ml)

To make:

1. In a small saucepan, warm the oil over low heat.

2. Add the chopped vanilla bean, cover, and allow to steep for 1 hour.

3. Remove from the heat and strain. It's all right if you see tiny brown specks in your oil. That's just the vanilla bean seeds — they're harmless. Save the vanilla bean for other uses.

4. Add the oil back to the pan and add the beeswax, cocoa butter, and lanolin and heat until just melted.

5. Remove from the heat and stir in essential oil if you desire. If left plain, it will smell like white chocolate, sweet and yummy!

To use: Scoop out approximately 1 teaspoon (5 ml), rub between your palms to warm and improve spreadability, then massage into each foot as necessary to keep them wonderfully moisturized and smooth.

Storage: Store in a 4-ounce (112 g) jar. No refrigeration is necessary. This butter may harden in cold weather, but will soften upon skin contact.

requires the attention of a doctor combined with a balanced, healthful diet and exercise.

Treatment: Treating the foot ailments of a diabetic is usually best left in the hands of a foot specialist — too many things could go awry if home treatment is attempted. There is one exception though: Foot specialists recommend using a good moisturizer on the feet daily to help keep any corns and calluses smooth and soft, thus heading off any potential infection caused by dry skin cracks. The Vanilla Foot Butter recipe above is one of my favorites.

Prevention: Prevention is key when dealing with diabetic feet. Here are some basic tips to remember:

- Inspect your feet daily for developing corns, calluses, blisters, or anything unusual such as color change, swelling, pain, or sores that are slow to heal. Treat minor corns and calluses immediately to prevent further development.
- Check shoes for fit and wear patterns and replace as necessary. They should never be too tight or too short, since this could further impair circulation. Never wear high heels or open-toed sandals.
- Wash your feet daily with a mild soap and warm water and make sure to completely dry between your toes. Using a blow dryer on the lowest setting does a super job of drying your feet. This is especially handy if your feet are tender and rubbing with a towel would cause discomfort. Dust with powder to keep perspiration in check.
- Don't go barefoot. Always wear shoes and loose seamless socks to avoid irritation.
- Keep feet soft by applying a thick cream every night.
- If you smoke, quit! I don't need to tell you that it contributes to poor circulation and poor health in general.
- Eat a well-balanced, high-fiber, low-fat diet.
- Finally, make exercise a daily habit.

See a Physician If: Diabetes is a serious disease and an ordinary foot problem should not be ignored; it could be life-threatening if not dealt with promptly. Attempting harsh home treatments such as cutting your calluses or corns could cause

In a pinch, you can use petroleum jelly or castor oil as softening foot treatments. If you'd like a product in an elegant tube to carry in your purse or stash in an office drawer, I recommend Elizabeth Arden's Eight Hour Cream. It's a bit expensive, but conveniently sized and doubles as an excellent lip gloss, cuticle conditioner, and nail buffing cream. It's been a popular product for many, many years.

bleeding and should **never** be performed. Even using a pumice stone too aggressively could open the gate for infection. Your best and safest bet is to visit a foot specialist.

DRY, CRACKED FEET

Causes: Dry skin can affect any part of the body, but the soles of your feet are very susceptible because they, like the palms of your hands, lack sebaceous (oil) glands to help keep them lubricated. These glands secrete sebum, which helps prevent the evaporation of moisture from the skin.

Years ago when I worked as an aesthetician and reflexologist in a salon, I observed many pairs of dry, cracked, scaly feet and was frequently asked to recommend or formulate a lotion or cream to aid in healing the condition. Dry skin can be the result of a nutritional deficiency (specifically vitamins A, B complex, C, D, or E) or just simple neglect. Rubbing lotion on your feet every day may help a bit, but basic foot care must become a daily habit.

Symptoms: I'm assuming that the dryness and cracks on your feet aren't caused by athlete's foot. If so, then treat accordingly. So that leaves us with neglect! If you ignore your feet and the types of shoes you stick them into, then an unpleasant situation can develop: rough, dry, sometimes painful, skin. Calluses can form on your heels, balls of your feet, and on your toes. They can thicken, then crack and harden if not pared down and softened. I've got a friend whose feet become so leatherlike and fissured in winter that sometimes she can barely walk because they hurt so much.

If you exercise, your feet perspire a lot. In the warmer months this does not pose a problem, but in winter, the air is drier and colder, and your soft, sweaty feet will dry and crack after removing your running shoes if you don't care for them properly.

Simply walking around barefoot a lot or wearing open-toed sandals can lead to dry skin on your feet. Your poor dogs need some type of barrier protection between you and the drying environment, be it lotion, cream, oil, or salve.

Treatment: If you've allowed your feet to become hard and leathery, you must first soften them before you can begin healing the dry skin condition. Try the Mineral Rich Oatmeal Soak on page 207 — it's very soothing!

Prevention: Don't wait until the dead of winter to start treating your painful, leathery feet; start at summer's end with some preventative maintenance so you never reach the dreaded skin-splitting stage.

See a Physician If: If the skin on your feet has become so hard, dry, and thick that it is resistant to home treatment, a foot specialist can file or pare down the buildup so you can then proceed with proper maintenance. If your feet have developed deep fissures, become inflamed, or bleed, see a doctor to prevent infection from setting in.

The elderly, in particular, often suffer from dry skin problems, mainly due to the inability to simply bend over and reach their feet to take care of them. A doctor or perhaps a nail technician would be of great help with basic foot care needs.

SUPER RICH, ALL-PURPOSE FOOT CREAM

Here's a recipe for the thickest cream I've ever made. It's got real staying power and will keep your feet the softest they've ever been. Guaranteed! It also doubles as a fantastic lip balm and dynamite cuticle conditioner.

3 tablespoons (45 ml) plus 1 teaspoon (5 ml) castor oil

2 teaspoons (10 ml) beeswax

15 drops peppermint essential oil

15 drops rosemary essential oil

Yield: approximately ¼ cup (60 ml)

To make:

1. Over very low heat, blend the castor oil and beeswax in a small saucepan, and heat until the wax is just melted. Remove from burner and allow to cool a bit.

2. Add the essential oil drops to the bottom of a 2-ounce (55 g) jar, then pour in the oil/wax mixture.

To use:

1. Apply enough of this wonderfully thick cream to your feet each night so that your ankles are covered as well. Put on socks.

2. In the morning, apply a dab to the dryest areas before getting dressed. I usually use this formula, or a similar one, every day or so for 8 months out of the year and find that from May through August a lighter cream will suffice.

MINERAL RICH OATMEAL SOAK

If you do this procedure every other day or so you will eventually and safely remove most of the hard skin on your feet and can then reduce the treatment to 2 times per week as maintenance. This footbath feels particularly good because of the oatmeal's moisturizing and softening properties.

1 footbath tub
½ cup (125 ml) very finely ground oatmeal
¼ cup (60 ml) white cosmetic clay
5 drops geranium, lavender, or eucalyptus essential oil (optional)
Pumice stone or foot file

Yield: 1 treatment

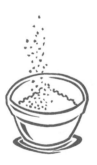

To make:

1. To make the ground oatmeal, put about ¾ cup (180 ml) old-fashioned "grocery store" variety oatmeal into a food processor and process until the oats are of a powderlike consistency.

2. Place a towel on the floor in front of the chair where you will be sitting as you soak your feet. Pour enough water into the tub (whatever temperature you desire) so that your ankles will be covered. Slowly stir in the oatmeal and clay until dissolved, then add essential oil if you desire.

To use:

1. Soak your feet for at least 10 to 15 minutes or until your calluses are soft, but not until your feet are "pruny."

2. Very gently scrub your calluses and/or corns with the pumice stone or file just until the top layer of tough dead skin has been removed.

3. Rinse, then roughly dry with a coarse towel.

4. Apply a heavy cream and put on socks.

Caution: Diabetics should not soak their feet. Most suffer from circulatory disorders and cannot feel if the water temperature is too hot or cold. Additionally, if the foot skin gets too soft as a result of soaking, it can lead to pre-ulcerations especially between the toes in the web spaces.

HEEL SPURS

Causes: The plantar fascia is a band of connective tissue that runs from the base of the heel to the base of the toes. Heel spurs begin when a partial separation occurs between this tissue and the heel bone. This injury may cause new bone growth in the affected area that projects out into the flesh of the foot. Other causes of heel spurs might be obesity, running, jogging, or jumping up and down in aerobics class, standing on your feet all day, wearing worn out shoes, and so forth. Anything that constantly strains the muscles that support your foot can lead to the formation of a spur.

Symptoms: A heel spur can feel like you have a rock permanently wedged in your heel or a painful bruise. The pain is most intense immediately after a period of rest, just when you begin to walk again. Actually, the more you walk, the better it feels, up to a point. Continued walking and long periods of standing will cause the heel to become quite tender.

Treatment: The painful inflammation in your heel needs to be relieved by resting your foot and applying heat with either a heating pad or hot water foot soaks to rev up the circulation, ease the pain, and reduce the swelling. When wearing shoes, place a half-inch-thick heel pad in your shoe to help cushion the pain and absorb shock. Arch supports may help to take some of the weight off your heel.

Prevention: Feet need to be stretched and allowed to relax throughout the day. If possible, remove your shoes several times a day and point and flex your feet for as long as you can and rotate your ankles. This relieves the pressure and tension on the plantar fascia.

By all means wear comfortable shoes. A firmer, motion-control shoe with a snug heel fit and ample padding in the heel area is recommended, especially if your job demands that you be on your feet a lot or you're an avid exerciser.

See a Physician If: If at-home therapy and heel padding doesn't help, your doctor may want to use steroid injections for temporary relief or may decide to make custom orthotics, which will redistribute your weight so that your foot is correctly balanced and the pressure is taken off the spur. As a last resort, your doctor can perform surgery to remove the spur (frequently this is done right in the office).

ANOTHER PAIN IN THE HEEL: CALCANEAL BUMPS

A calcaneal bump or Haglund's deformity (or "pump bump" as it is sometimes called) is a bony protuberance or enlargement behind your heel where the Achilles tendon attaches to the bone. "It bothers mostly women, especially around the ripe old age of 22," says Walter J. Pedowitz, M.D. "This is about the age when the sneaker-wearing college student suddenly enters the corporate world and starts wearing heels to work." The deformity is caused by increased friction of the heel against the hard shoe counter, which leads to irritation. Eventually a bursal sac (a fluid-filled "cushion") forms on the bump. This sac can then get inflamed and painful. Mule-style shoes or slingbacks are recommended to avoid pressure on the heel.

HOT FEET

Causes: There are lots of causes for hot feet, such as stress, anxiety, insufficient water intake, walking barefoot on hot pavement or beach sand, shoes and socks that are too heavy for the season, or standing all day.

Symptoms: Having hot feet is not a serious threat to your health, just a nuisance. If your feet are hot, then usually so is the rest of you, and uncomfortable to boot! Many times the symptom of hot feet is combined with itchiness, profuse sweating, and/or odor, but we'll address those individually later. I just want to show you how you can bring relief to your fiery feet and cool the rest of your body simultaneously.

Treatment: My very active eighty-seven-year-old grandfather tends a large garden and raises cattle. I think his only complaints in life are his weather-sensitive, arthritic knees and his hot feet. Georgia summers can get quite sultry, so he cools his feet by soaking them daily in cool water and adds a few spoonfuls of his favorite medicinal footbath powder that contains camphor and eucalyptus. (Then he promptly falls asleep!) You could try this too, but instead of powder, add a few drops each of camphor, eucalyptus, and peppermint essential oils.

Prevention: Here are a few tips to help keep your feet cool and fresh at all times:

◆ Wash feet at least once but maybe twice a day with cool water, using a peppermint or tea tree essential oil soap. Try September's Sun Herbal Soap Company's "Mad about Mint" or "Tea Tree Foot Soap" (see Resources). Don't forget to dry between your toes.

◆ Use a mint or menthol-based foot powder liberally morning and night to keep feet delightfully dry.

◆ Wear comfortable, roomy shoes with light, airy socks so feet can breathe.

◆ Drink plenty of water.

◆ If you must stand all day, try to slip off your shoes every hour or so and prop your feet up. If that's not possible, remove your shoes and simply wiggle your toes and rotate your ankles for a bit of exercise.

◆ Take your shoes, socks, and/or hosiery off as soon as you get home and go barefoot for the rest of the evening if you can. Feet need to feel the cool ground beneath them for as many hours as possible each day.

See a Physician If: If your feet are not cooling down by using any of the above treatments and are hot *and* itchy, rashy, or developing dry skin cracks, you should probably visit a foot specialist to rule out athlete's foot, an allergy, or a rash like poison oak/ivy.

FOOT FACT

The average temperature inside your shoes is 106°F. It's a wonder your feet don't just quit and go on strike!

ROSEMARY AND PEPPERMINT
COOLING LEG AND FOOT GEL

A couple of years ago, I created a fabulous herbal gel formula to use as a facial cleanser for dry, sensitive skin. It occurred to me while writing this section that it could double as a super cooling leg and foot gel, too. It leaves legs and feet feeling comfortably cool and moisturized. Contrary to what you might think, it leaves minimal residue and sinks right in. It's excellent to use after shaving your legs.

1 teaspoon (5 ml) finely powdered marsh mallow root

1 tablespoon (15 ml) water

2 drops peppermint essential oil

2 drops rosemary or eucalyptus essential oil

Yield: 1 treatment

To make: In a small bowl, stir together all ingredients until a tan-colored, thick, speckled, slippery gel forms. This will happen very quickly.

To use: Apply 1 teaspoon (5 ml) of this gel to each leg and foot and massage in until the gel is no longer slippery.

Storage: Cover and refrigerate any leftovers for up to 3 days.

Note: To make the gel especially refreshing, chill for 1 hour prior to use.

ON YOUR FEET ALL DAY: A CAREER TIP

In 1987, while in school training for my aesthetician license, my instructors stressed this point over and over again, "Give your feet a few minutes' daily care. It's essential to good posture and good health. Healthy feet help produce a more pleasing personality."

Initially, I didn't understand how taking care of my feet affected my personality. After I'd worked in a salon for a while, it became clear. Standing eight hours a day in fashionable shoes hurts! Anyone who works on his or her feet all day knows that if your feet are constantly hurting, you feel miserable. It's much easier to smile and be cheerful with comfortable, cared-for feet.

MINT CHILLER FOOT LOTION

You've probably seen, if not used, the popular pink peppermint foot lotions sold by a few bath and body shops located in malls nationwide. They usually sell for approximately twenty dollars for a 16-ounce (448 g) bottle. That seems pretty pricey to me! Here's how to make your own for a fraction of the price. Mine smells more invigorating and minty, too, and it's super refreshing!

½ cup (125 ml) almond or soybean oil

1 tablespoon (15 ml) beeswax

½ teaspoon (2.5 ml) borax

⅓ cup (80 ml) plus 1 tablespoon (15 ml) warm, strong peppermint tea

3 drops red or green food coloring (optional)

½ teaspoon (2.5 ml) peppermint or spearmint essential oil

Yield: 1 cup (250 ml)

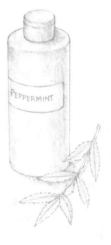

To make:

1. In a small pan over very low heat, melt the oil and wax.

2. In another saucepan, stir the borax into the warm tea until completely dissolved, and add food coloring if desired. (The peppermint tea can be made by simply pouring a cup of boiling water over a peppermint tea bag or 1 teaspoon [5 ml] of the dried herb, steeping for 5 to 10 minutes, then straining and cooling a bit.)

3. The two mixtures should be approximately the same temperature before you perform the next step. While whisking vigorously with your small whisk, slowly drizzle the warm tea/borax liquid into the oil/wax mixture, then add the essential oil. The cream will begin to thicken and should have a lotion-like consistency. If you place the oil/wax pan in a bowl of ice while whisking, the lotion will set up much faster.

To use: Massage into legs and feet anytime they need a little revitalizing. Keep the lotion in the refrigerator in the summer for an extra chilling sensation!

Storage: Store in a plastic squeeze bottle or decorative glass bottle. Use within thirty days, or sooner if weather is hot.

INGROWN TOENAILS

Causes: Ingrown toenails are nails that have become imbedded in the surrounding soft flesh of the toe. The big toe is most often affected, but the other toes can also suffer.

This painful condition can be caused by wearing short, tight shoes, socks, or hosiery; poor nail care; injury to the nail bed; fungus; and heredity. Obese people are particularly susceptible, too. Their feet gain weight just like the rest of the body and the skin can swell up and around the toenail. Combine this with the excess pressure placed upon the feet, and a bit of improper nail clipping, and you've got a recipe for pain.

Most ingrown toenails are self-inflicted. If you rip off your toenails with your fingers instead of cutting them, you leave jagged edges, which dig into the nail groove when your tight shoe presses against the toenail. Improper clipping by cutting the nail too short and rounding the corners can cause the same problem.

> **FOOT FACT**
>
> Ten percent of Americans have had an ingrown toenail at one time or another. It is the most common toenail impairment.

Symptoms: An infection called *paronychia* can result when the toenail penetrates the flesh. It begins as minor swelling, redness, and clear fluid oozing from the site. If ignored, it can become infected, very painful and swollen. Walking at this point is unbearable. If still left untreated, pus will exude from the infected site and red streaks can appear along the foot and shoot up the leg. The infection is dangerous now and can enter the bloodstream, causing you to become ill, possibly leading to the loss of a toe, foot, or leg if gangrene sets in. This, thankfully, is a rare occurrence.

Treatment: To treat an ingrown toenail in its beginning stages, soak your foot in a foot tub filled with warm, strong sage and yarrow tea (make this by using ¼ cup [60 ml] of each dried herb per gallon of boiling water, then steep, strain, and cool until comfortable), ½ cup (125 ml) of sea salt, and a few drops of tea tree or lavender essential oil for 10 to 15 minutes. Dry thoroughly. Now, take a sliver of cotton and using a toothpick, ever so gently wedge the cotton under the offending toenail. Leave it there until the nail grows out. It will help direct the nail's growth over the skin. Apply a drop of thyme, lavender, or tea tree essential oil on the site daily to help keep infection at bay.

Prevention: Try these tips to help prevent the occurrence of this painful affliction:

- Clip toenails straight across so that they are just about even with the tip of the toe and file any pointed edges smooth with an emery board.
- Examine your feet daily after washing and drying to nip any potential problems in the bud.
- Wear comfortable shoes and socks. Shoes and/or hosiery should never constrict your feet.

See a Physician If: If you're diabetic, don't allow a minor foot malady to become potentially life-threatening; see a foot specialist immediately. For an infection, antibiotics may be prescribed to clear it up. If an ingrown toenail is a recurrent problem, your doctor may want to perform a *matrixectomy* (removal of the germinal matrix, the source of nail growth, along with the edge of the nail plate). This is a permanent narrowing of the toenail.

FOOT FACT

Ingrown toenails most often occur in children, teens, and young adults, primarily because they don't heed early warning signs that something is amiss. Also, young people's feet grow so fast that they frequently wear shoes that are too short, tight, or worn out, which puts pressure and friction on the edges of the toenails. Foot health is not uppermost in their thoughts at this age either. Toenails are often not cut properly and feet are basically neglected. This is why it's essential that you examine your child's feet every day and instill the importance of proper foot care.

ODORIFEROUS AND SWEATY FEET

Causes: Think back a few decades ago (depending on your age) to Halloween night. Do you remember running up to the neighbor's door, all dressed up in your scariest costume, and yelling, "Trick or treat, smell my feet, give me something good to eat?" I realize it was all said in jest, but I can guarantee your neighbors wouldn't find that such a "treat" if you really made them smell your feet! All kidding aside, foot odor, or plantar bromidrosis, can be a seriously embarrassing physical as well as psychological problem for some people. It is caused by an overabundance of foot perspiration and bacteria.

The rate of sweat production is greatly affected by a wide range of emotions such as fear, nervousness, falling in love, and performance anxiety, be it sexual or on-the-job stress. Drinking lots of water, exercising heavily, working at a physically demanding job, or wearing tight-fitting shoes or shoes made of nonbreathable materials for extended periods of time will also cause your feet to sweat. Some people have a genetic predisposition to foot odor and wetness, which tends to run in families.

Symptoms: When moisture and bacteria comingle inside a pair of shoes, they can create such an overwhelming stench that the poor sufferer will avoid social occasions and even shopping for new shoes. Excessive perspiration will cause destruction of footwear as the stitching, construction materials, and padding breakdown prematurely from the constant pressure and moisture within.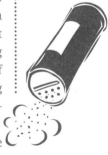

Foot odor is "unique and, next to alcoholic breath, may be the most distinctive scent in the office setting. It's often described as musty, amino-like, cheesy, or rancid," says Walter J. Pedowitz, M.D.

Treatment: You know when your feet stink, unless you suffer from odor perception deficit. There are people who actually can't discern a sweet fragrance from stink (poor souls) and some who have gotten so used to the way their feet smell that they no longer notice the unpleasantness, but everyone around them does! Hopefully, if you suffer from this smelly affliction you will try some of my remedies to fix this distressful, air-fouling problem.

Prevention: Follow these tips for fresh feet:

- First and foremost, wash and dry your feet once or twice daily. Proper hygiene is imperative!
- Increase your chlorophyll intake. Spirulina, parsley, and green drinks are high in vitamin A and chlorophyll, which is a known internal odor fighter.
- Alternate shoes each day to allow for a 24-hour dry out period between wearings.
- Sprinkle baking soda into your shoes after you take them off for the evening to help absorb moisture and odor.
- If you're prone to foot odor, avoid strong foods such as garlic, onions, certain cheeses, black pepper, and eggs.
- Wear baking soda impregnated, cushioned insoles in your shoes and change them often.
- Make sure hose, shoes, and socks are made of natural fibers, fit properly, and allow your feet to breathe.
- Change socks or hosiery twice a day if necessary and reapply powder to keep feet super dry and prevent soggy skin.
- Underarm antiperspirant can be applied to the soles of your feet as well. It works for some people by lessening the amount of sweat produced and preventing bacterial growth. If you'd like to try this approach, I recommend using a natural brand first. Health food stores carry various herbal-based brands sans chemicals.

See a Physician If: If your condition is not responding to any of the above measures, a foot specialist may want to administer a topical antibiotic or recommend daily soaks with potassium permanganate to decrease odor production. Other drugs such as tranquilizers to soothe a nervous disposition or topical scented formaldehyde can be prescribed, but can have terrible side effects and should be avoided if at all possible. Diseases such as hyperthyroidism, hypoadrenalism, anemia, and thermoregulatory disturbances can cause profuse sweating, too, and should be ruled out.

ODOR AWAY REFRESHING FOOT SPRAY

1 cup (250 ml) commer-
   cial witch hazel or ½
   cup (125 ml) of your
   homemade witch hazel
   tincture added to ½
   cup (125 ml) distilled
   water
20 drops spearmint or
   peppermint essential oil
40 drops geranium essen-
   tial oil

Yield: 1 cup (250 ml)

To make: Pour all ingredients into an 8-ounce decorative spray bottle. Shake well.
To use: Spray feet any time they need cooling and revitalizing. Best to use if you're not going to be wearing shoes for the next hour or so, so feet can dry naturally. This allows the astringent properties of the witch hazel and the cooling, deodorizing, and antimicrobial properties of the essential oils to go about their duties.
Storage: Refrigeration is not necessary. Use within one year for maximum potency.

WHITE OAK REMEDY

The following remedy was actually recommended in 1883 by J. I. Lighthall, the Great Indian Medicine Man, in his book, *The Indian Household Medicine Guide.* "There is no tree better known than the White Oak, nor is there a tree more useful to mankind. It grows in all parts of the United States. There are three kinds of Oaks: the red, the white, and the black. The inner bark is the part used as a medicine, and a very good one it is, too.

"**Medicinal properties and uses:** The bark is a powerful astringent. It makes a splendid wash for old sores and wounds when mattering and not inclined to heal. The best form to use it in is a strong tea made from the green bark. It will cure bad smelling and sweaty feet by washing them with it."

ODOR NEUTRALIZING ORANGE FOOT POWDER

Foot odor has more than just one symptom. It is frequently accompanied by soggy skin, blisters, tenderness between the toes, and susceptibility to fungus and infection. This powder will help to absorb the odor, keep your feet dry, and fight fungus (if you add the tea tree and thyme essential oils or geranium essential oil). Orange essential oil is a terrific odor fighter!

½ cup (125 ml) baking soda
½ cup (125 ml) arrowroot
2 tablespoons (30 ml) zinc oxide powder
2 tablespoons (30 ml) fine, white clay
1 teaspoon (5 ml) orange or geranium essential oil (both do a great job!)
½ teaspoon (2.5 ml) tea tree essential oil (optional)
½ teaspoon (2.5 ml) thyme essential oil (optional)

Yield: approximately 1¼ cups (310 ml)

To make: Mix dry ingredients in a large bowl or food processor. Add the essential oils a few drops at a time and thoroughly incorporate into powder.

To use: Sprinkle into shoes and socks once or twice daily.

Storage: Store this in a special shaker container or recycle a plastic spice jar (not one that previously held dried onions or garlic, though). Refrigeration is not necessary. Use within one year for maximum potency.

PLANTAR WARTS

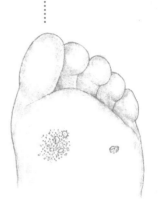

Causes: A *verruca plantaris*, or plantar wart, appears on the plantar surface or sole of your foot and is caused by an easily transmittable virus. You can just as easily transmit it to other parts of your body or to someone else. Just like athlete's foot fungus, the virus can be contracted by walking barefoot in warm, moist environments such as in gyms, locker rooms, saunas, showers, pool areas, and public bathrooms. Cracks or abrasions on your feet are an open invitation for the virus to go deep inside the dermal layers and take up residence. Scratching or shaving over the affected area can also spread the infection.

Plantar
warts

Symptoms: The wart can range in size from a tiny dot to the size of a nickel or larger and appear singly or in clusters, but can easily be confused with a callus or corn because the warts are covered with thick skin tissue. A plantar wart, though, has a distinct black or brown pinpoint in the center, which is the site of a blood vessel, and will hurt if you squeeze it and bleed if you cut it; a corn will not. These warts occur most frequently on the balls and heels of the feet.

Plantar warts can be quite painful and become pushed deep inside the skin due to weight and shoe pressure.

A mosaic wart is caused by the same virus, is irregular in shape and bleeds easily when irritated, and can eventually form a large cluster of a hundred or more tiny warts. This patch of warts can cover the entire bottom of the foot and has a rougher, thicker surface than a plantar wart.

Treatment: A cure for these pesky, painful growths can be elusive at best because they frequently go away spontaneously and also tend to recur spontaneously in the same areas. There is no guaranteed cure, natural or chemical. Just when you think they're gone, here they come again.

FOOT FACT

The American Podiatric Medical Association says that, "Children, especially teenagers, tend to be more susceptible to warts than adults; some people seem to be immune, and never get them."

Some foot specialists recommend the cost-effective treatment of repeatedly applying salicylic acid drops (found in the foot care section of your drugstore). File the wart down slightly with an emery board daily, apply a drop of acid, file again the next day, apply acid . . . keep treating daily for several weeks or months until the wart dissolves. Care should be taken to avoid getting this acid on the surrounding skin, as it can burn and dissolve healthy tissue as well as the wart(s).

Caution: Diabetics should never try this.

Herbal and folklore wart remedies abound. You could try applying the milky, sticky sap from a dandelion stem, calendula stem, or milkweed stem to the wart and covering with an adhesive bandage. Change dressing daily. These saps act as corrosive agents to remove the wart.

Tea tree essential oil can be applied "neat" (undiluted), as can garlic oil. These both have powerful antiviral properties. A slice of raw garlic can be taped to the affected area with a fresh piece being applied daily. Vitamin A oil is said to remove warts, too. No one treatment works for everyone. Whatever method you choose to try, keep at it. Warts can be stubborn creatures.

Prevention: Since the virus that causes plantar warts is highly contagious, please avoid going barefoot in the gym or around swimming pools, or any place that's public, warm, and moist. Wash and dry your feet daily and put powder in your shoes to absorb moisture. Also, if you are treating or inspecting someone else's infected feet, wear disposable gloves and wash your hands thoroughly.

See a Physician If: Plantar warts are sometimes difficult to treat. If yours continue to spread and are making walking painful, see a doctor. Electric needle treatments, acid peels, freezing with dry ice, or laser surgery can be used by a foot specialist to get rid of warts. Try to avoid surgery if possible so that no painful scars are left on the bottom of your foot.

SORE, ACHY FEET

Causes: You probably know the cause of your sore feet. Perhaps you stand all day at work, chase your children around the house, wear fashionable shoes that don't fit properly, or work out a lot. Whatever the cause, you want relief and you want it now!

Symptoms: Sore feet feel tired, like they've lost their "spring." Sometimes they even swell, burn, or feel tender if you've been wearing snug-fitting, blister-causing shoes.

Treatment: The following recipes will revitalize your sore, achy dogs. They serve double duty in that they also reduce foot odor.

The following two quotes are from the book *Herbal Recipes* by Clarence Meyer (Meyerbooks, Glenwood, Illinois, 1978). It's interesting to see the remedies that were prescribed nearly two centuries ago for foot problems.

"The bark of the root of bittersweet with chamomile and wormwood makes an ointment of great value, which is an excellent thing for a bruise, sprain, calice, swelling, or for corns" (*New Guide to Health: or, Botanic Physician,* Samuel Thomson, 1831).

"Take tansy, wormwood, horehound, catnip, and hops, of each an equal quantity. Bruise them and put them into a kettle, cover over with spirits and lard, and let it stand 2 weeks; then simmer awhile and strain. Add 1 lb. of common white turpentine to every 10 lbs. of the ointment. This ointment is very cooling, resolvent, relaxing, and emollient. It is very useful in sprains, contusions, swellings, dislocations, contracted sinews, etc." (*The American Practice of Medicine,* W. Beach, M.D., 1833).

Prevention: Sometimes daily sore feet can't be completely prevented due to job or lifestyle demands. But by wearing really comfortable shoes with shock-absorbing insoles; massaging your feet; taking soothing herbal footbaths made with yarrow, sage, thyme, or peppermint with a scoop of baking soda and Epsom salts added; and paying extra attention to foot hygiene, you should have lots of spring in your step most of the time.

See a Physician If: If your feet are chronically sore, and changing your shoe environment and trying the Sweet Relief — Aspirin for the Feet Salve (page 222) treatment doesn't help alleviate some of the soreness, then see a foot specialist. He or she may want to check for misalignment problems, ingrown toenails, arthritis, bunion development, and so forth.

SWEET RELIEF — ASPIRIN FOR THE FEET SALVE

This recipe calls for St.-John's-wort oil. To make the infused oil, see Julie Bailey's Calendula Blossom Oil recipe on page 192, but substitute St.–John's–wort flowers for the calendula blossoms. Fresh is best, but dried is okay. You can also purchase the prepared oil in better health food stores. All of the herbs in this recipe have pain-relieving properties.

½ cup (125 ml) St.-John's-wort oil

1 tablespoon (15 ml) dried meadowsweet or 2 tablespoons (30 ml) fresh flowers and leaves (wilted for 24 hours in the shade to remove excess moisture)

1 tablespoon (15 ml) powdered white willow bark

½ teaspoon (2.5 ml) powdered cayenne pepper

1–2 tablespoons (15–30 ml) beeswax (use the greater amount if you want a stiffer salve)

10 drops each peppermint, camphor, eucalyptus, and clove essential oils

Yield: approximately ½ cup (125 ml)

To make:

1. In a half-pint, widemouthed jar, combine the St.-John's-wort oil, meadowsweet, white willow, and cayenne. Tightly seal and place in the full sun for approximately 4 weeks.

2. Shake daily.

3. Strain through hosiery or cheesecloth to remove the powder granules. Make sure to squeeze all the oil out of the straining material to get every precious drop.

4. In a small saucepan, over very low heat, melt the beeswax and stir in oil. Remove from heat and add essential oils after mixture cools a bit.

5. Pour into a decorative widemouthed plastic or glass jar.

To use: Massage a fingerful of salve into clean, tired feet as desired. This feels especially good if you can talk someone else into doing the massaging for you!

Storage: Refrigeration is not necessary. Use within six months for maximum potency.

TOENAIL FUNGUS

Causes: Ugly and embarrassing — that's how best to describe the condition of toenails infected with fungus. People with toenail fungus often avoid social situations that call for baring their feet, such as pool parties or strolling on the beach.

Onychomycosis is caused by microorganisms called dermatophytes, which are similar to those that cause athlete's foot. These organisms are present on your clothes and in your shoes, the gym, and even your organically fortified garden soil. They're practically unavoidable.

Symptoms: One or more of your toenails will begin to look a bit abnormal. Color changes can appear, such as long, yellowish streaks or white patches that can be scraped off. The nail can lift and begin to separate from the nail bed, thicken, and become brittle and flaky. It can also become distorted in shape and begin to twist. This fungus can be transmitted easily to your fingernails, or to other members of your family for that matter, if you constantly pick at your toes without washing your hands afterward. It sounds disgusting, but lots of people do it unintentionally.

Treatment: In order to treat toenail fungus, you have to get underneath the nail, which can be difficult. The fungus lives on the soft skin of the nail bed. The herbs and oils in the recipes on pages 224 and 225 have traditionally been used by herbalists with much success if applied at least once a day. Twice is better.

Prevention: Since toenail fungus is infectious, take the same precautions as you would with athlete's foot and wear the appropriate footwear when in public bathing places. Observe proper daily foot hygiene; keep feet fresh and dry with powder and clean changes of socks/hosiery; wear good-fitting, breathable shoes; and never trim toenails too close to the skin or cut the skin.

See a Physician If: Toenail fungus is difficult to treat. If the above measures fail, visit your foot specialist. He or she may want to prescribe a topical or oral medication to combat the fungus or perhaps remove the diseased nail, depending on the severity of the infection. Medications are not without side effects, and do not always work, either.

ANTIFUNGAL TOENAIL LINIMENT

4 tablespoons (60 ml) dried black walnut hulls or 8 tablespoons (120 ml) fresh and chopped fine

2 tablespoons (30 ml) dried, chopped goldenseal or Oregon grape root

1 tablespoon (15 ml) powdered myrrh gum

40 drops tea tree essential oil

40 drops thyme essential oil

40 drops tincture of iodine

2 cups (500 ml) vodka, brandy, rum, or gin (must be at least 80-proof or 40 percent alcohol by volume)

Yield: approximately 1½ cups (375 ml)

To make:

1. In a quart-sized (liter-sized), wide-mouthed canning jar, add the black walnut hulls, goldenseal, myrrh gum, essential oils, and iodine, then pour in the alcohol. Cap tightly and store in a dark, cool place.

2. Shake daily.

3. After at least 14 days have passed (I recommend 4 to 12 weeks; it makes for a stronger formula), you may strain the mixture through hosiery-lined cheesecloth, then squeeze and twist the cloth to wring out all the liquid.

4. Pour the finished formula into two, 8-ounce (228-g) bottles with dropper tops.

To use: Morning, noon, and night, if possible, apply a few drops to toenails, rub in thoroughly, and allow to dry before putting on hosiery, socks, or footwear. Repeat this procedure daily for as long as it takes to rid your toenails of fungus. The herbs in this recipe have potent antifungal and antimicrobial properties.

Storage: Refrigeration is not necessary. This product will keep indefinitely!

TOUGH ON FUNGUS TOENAIL DROPS

You can use this recipe in conjunction with the Antifungal Toenail Liniment on the previous page. Apply this oil after the liniment has dried. Use this oil consistently for at least six months or longer or until the fungus has disappeared.

2 teaspoons (10 ml) tea tree essential oil
2 teaspoons (10 ml) thyme essential oil
2 teaspoons (10 ml) camphor essential oil
1 1-ounce (28 g) dropper-topped bottle

Yield: approximately 1 ounce (28 g)

To make: Combine all three essential oils and pour into the bottle. Shake well.

To use: Place a drop or two on each toenail morning and night and rub in well, then dress as you normally do.

Storage: Store in a cool, dry place.

FOOT FACT

Foot specialists estimate that approximately seven to eight million people in the United States suffer from toenail fungus, but only a quarter of them seek a doctor for treatment.

PART IV:
SOOTHING SKIN CARE

Tips and Techniques
for a Lifetime of Radiant Skin

Stephanie L. Tourles

INTRODUCTION

"Smoother, younger-looking skin in seven days. Guaranteed or your money back." How many times have you fallen for that marketing ploy? Most cosmetic companies are very adept at knowing which buttons to push to entice you to purchase their merchandise and empty your wallet, in a flash, with promises of restored youth. The department store counters beckon with their glamorous posters, beautifully made-up salespeople, and buy-one-get-one-free offers. These companies prey on your emotions, all in the guise of making you look and feel better about yourself.

The cosmetics and bodycare industry is made up of many multimillion-dollar corporations. They are in business to make money, and indeed they do. Skin care products have one of the highest price mark-ups of any commodity on the market. Don't get me wrong, though — there are some companies whose products actually do produce the desired results and whose prices are not overly inflated. You will generally find their skin care wares in better health food stores or from a salon or spa that puts a strong emphasis on premium natural ingredients in the products they represent.

It's my belief that an educated consumer is a discerning consumer. In this book, I hope to educate you as to what constitutes a good versus a bad cosmetic. You'll learn about skin form and function, its needs, and how those needs can be met by various herbs, oils, and other natural ingredients. You'll be armed with the knowledge of what to look for in a commercial product as well as how to make your own formulas.

It's only natural to want to look your best, to make a positive, lasting impression upon the people that you greet. When you look good, you feel good. You project an air of confidence. When you are dissatisfied with your appearance, your self-esteem suffers.

Ever had a day when it's an absolute must that you look super for an important event, only to have an unexpected blemish appear in the middle of your forehead or on the tip of your nose, or have a rash develop on your neck? Your skin doesn't always cooperate the way you want it to — especially when you want it to. It reacts to emotional upheavals, stress, weather, makeup, dirt, grease, food, and hormones. Remember the Murphy's Law of skin care: If something can flare up, it will . . . and at the most inopportune time!

When your skin looks good, it's translucent, luminous, radiant, and simply exudes glowing health. When it's behaving badly, it's upsetting and occasionally disfiguring, resulting in acne scars, scaly patches, broken capillaries, puffiness, rashes, eczema, or warts. Your potentially beautiful skin can become downright unattractive and ugly from lack of "sun sense." Accumulated sun exposure, over the years, will produce a slew of leathery wrinkles and age spots, which in and of themselves are depressing, but additionally, the incidence of skin cancer is rapidly on the rise. It's not pretty and can be fatal.

This section takes a holistic approach to skin care: Health within is reflected by beautiful skin without. I'll show you how to integrate nutrition, stress reduction, and herbs and other natural ingredients to help systemically remedy your skin care concerns, instead of merely treating the exterior symptoms as is the common approach. Combine this knowledge with a proper cleansing routine and sound sun protection and you'll have the recipe for a lifetime of fabulous looking skin.

— Stephanie L. Tourles

CHAPTER 12
Skin Care Basics

▼▼▼

Caring for your skin doesn't have to be a complicated affair. It's quite simple, actually — just don't tell the salespeople behind the department store cosmetics counter I said that. Their livelihood depends on the number of bottles of skin-pampering potions you purchase. If they had their way, you'd be buying an eye cream, a lip exfoliating cream, a lip gloss, a lipstick sealer, a throat cream, a diuretic for the puffiness under your eyes, under-eye circle concealer, antiwrinkle cream, skin-lightening lotion, body sloughing cream, bust-enhancing cream, thigh cream, a blackhead/pore-tightening mask, youth serum (once they get it figured out), pre-cleanser, regular cleanser, clarifying lotion, hyperpigmentation spot treatment cream — the list is endless.

Cosmetic companies want to sell you hope in a jar, the hope of fresh, new, wrinkle-free skin and restored youth. Let's face it — it's never going to happen! However, your quest for a vibrant, healthy appearance needn't be terribly expensive or complicated or include a bevy of synthetic chemicals. In this chapter, I'll show you how to identify your skin type and discuss what products are most beneficial. You'll learn how to get down to the basics of simple but effective natural skin care.

KEEP IT SIMPLE

Chapter 1 detailed how nutrition, exercise, sunlight, water consumption, and sleep are vital to a healthy body and clear skin. These factors affect us internally and result in vibrant and glowing skin fortified from the inside out. Your skin must be properly cared for externally as well, but this doesn't mean you have to spend hundreds of dollars every year on the latest synthetic technological skin care breakthrough, or even sixty dollars on a tiny jar of throat firming cream with encapsulated liposomes that burst upon your skin at scheduled intervals.

I believe in a basic skin care routine. Five products — a cleanser, a toner or astringent, a moisturizer, an exfoliant or antioxidant, and a sunscreen — are all anyone, man or woman, needs to use to maintain healthy skin. Find a moisturizing sunscreen, and the number drops to four. Doesn't get much simpler than that!

- **Cleanser** — to wash away dirt, makeup, toxins, and pollutants
- **Toner or astringent** — to remove any residual cleanser or oil from the skin and to temporarily refine the appearance of large pores
- **Moisturizer** — to replenish and minimize wear and tear
- **Exfoliator or antioxidant** — to refresh and smooth the complexion, such as a gentle facial scrub, alpha- or beta-hydroxy gel or cream, or topical vitamin C
- **Sunscreen** — to protect

TOP FOUR CLEANSING TIPS

1. If you wear foundation, powder, or waterproof face and eye makeup, be sure to cleanse your skin twice. The first cleansing removes the makeup, and the second cleansing removes excess sebum, and dead skin, and deep cleans your pores.

2. Rinse, rinse, rinse. You can never rinse your face and body too much! Cleansing products, massage oil, makeup, and soap can leave a film on your skin that will clog pores.

3. No matter how oily your complexion, limit your cleansing routine to twice a day, to avoid stripping your skin's protective acid mantle.

4. Avoid hot water! Hot water dehydrates and irritates most skin types. Use tepid or warm water only.

DISCOVERING YOUR SKIN TYPE

Granted, maintaining a healthy lifestyle is key to having beautiful skin, but the real secret to having skin that is irresistible to touch and behold is to accurately know your skin type and care for it accordingly. Too many people treat their skin with the wrong products; instead of improving the condition of their skin, they actually worsen it.

To help you identify and evaluate your skin type and understand its special needs, seven different classifications are detailed below. Nine times out of ten you will fall into one of these categories, but some of you may overlap into another category or two. That's okay. Everybody's unique.

Oily Skin

Characteristics: Medium-to-large pores in T-zone area and perhaps on the cheeks, shoulders, neck, chest, and back as well. Overactive sebaceous glands give the skin a slick, shiny appearance within an hour after cleansing. May or may not be prone to acne or pimples, but pores do become clogged easily. Oily skin is not prone to fine lines and wrinkles because it is well-lubricated.

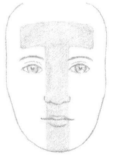

Seasonal Variations: Heat and humidity tend to increase the amount of sebum production whereas cooler temperatures and lower humidity are a boon for oily complexions. Surface dehydration (lack of moisture) may occur in very cold, dry weather.

The area of the face that encompasses the forehead, nose, and chin is known as the T-zone.

Cleansing: Use a water-based gel, milk, or clay cleanser that does not dry out the skin's surface twice a day. You may use a gentle, herbal glycerin or goat milk soap if you wish, as long as it does not dry out your skin. Your goal here is to remove the excess oil, but not strip your skin of its protective barrier. "Squeaky clean" is not what you're after! (If your skin is extremely oily, you may need to bathe your body twice a day, using your preferred cleanser.)

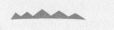

SKINFORMATION

Overdrying the surface of an oily complexion, it is believed, may stimulate the sebaceous glands to produce more oil — exactly the opposite of what you are trying to achieve!

Toning: A gentle, astringent herbal tea such as yarrow, sage, or peppermint will remove any leftover cleanser and dirt from the facial skin. Avoid using isopropyl (rubbing) alcohol; it's too harsh and extremely drying. If you tend to break out or have excessively oily skin on your shoulders, neck, chest, or back, you may want to apply an herbal astringent tea to those areas as often as necessary to remove the oil and freshen your skin.

Moisturizing: Depending on the degree of oiliness, you may not need a moisturizer at all or at the very least, use a light moisturizing aloe vera–based spray or aromatic hydrosol to keep the facial skin's surface hydrated. Apply a light moisturizing lotion to your body if you feel it's needed.

Special Treatments: Use of a clay mask or exfoliating scrub twice a week will discourage formation of blackheads, minimize breakouts, and reduce the appearance of enlarged pores. Alpha- or beta-hydroxy acid treatments, used twice a week, are good to smooth and refine the skin's surface (these products can also be used on oily areas of the body). An herbal facial steam using yarrow, sage, or rosemary with a couple of drops of tea tree essential oil is perfect for disinfecting any minor pimples or open blemishes you may have. For pimples, I recommend an overnight spot treatment mask using 2 to 3 drops of tea tree or thyme (chemotype linalol) essential oil combined with a bit of clay and water to help heal those pesky blemishes. *Note:* Do not use a facial scrub if you have acne, as this can further aggravate the condition.

Normal Skin

Characteristics: Neither too dry nor too oily. Usually free of blemishes, but may form blackheads. May get a little oily in T-zone 4 to 6 hours after cleansing depending on humidity and temperature. Pores are normal in size.

Seasonal Variations: The face tends to be oilier in summer than winter and the entire body may suffer from surface dehydration in very cold weather.

Cleansing: For the face, use a gentle water- or milk-based cleanser that will remove surface impurities without stripping skin of oil twice a day. You can use the same cleanser for your body or a mild natural soap.

Toning: Lavender, rose, rosemary, German chamomile, or orange floral waters refresh and further cleanse the skin.

Moisturizing: A light but protective lotion designed to seal in moisture is recommended for both the face and the body. Avoid anything too heavy as it will cause oiliness.

Special Treatments: For the face, a pore-refining clay mask once a week or a moisturizing mask in winter can be used if necessary. Alpha- or beta-hydroxy acid treatments are recommended twice a week to minimize fine lines and smooth the skin. An herbal facial steam once a week helps cleanse pores.

Dry Skin

Characteristics: Lacks natural oil and moisture, the basic requirements for that healthy glow! May appear flaky or scaly and be rough textured if very dry. Has small pores and feels taut after cleansing. Develops lines and wrinkles more rapidly than any other skin type. Ages prematurely.

Seasonal Variations: Dry skin loves warm temperatures and humidity, but the winter can be a challenge. Cold temperatures and dry air rob the skin of moisture resulting in chapping, irritation, and redness.

Cleansing: For the face, use a moisture-rich cleansing milk or cream twice a day. Avoid soap at all costs. Products enriched with chamomile, calendula, or lavender are nurturing and gentle for this skin type. For your body, I recommend cleansing with a small drawstring bath bag filled with oatmeal. Once wet, the oatmeal will cover your skin with moisturizing "oat milk," which is quite soothing for dry skin.

Toning: The classic rosewater and glycerin lotion makes a perfect toner to rehydrate and further cleanse thirsty facial skin.

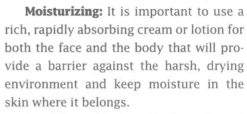
Moisturizing: It is important to use a rich, rapidly absorbing cream or lotion for both the face and the body that will provide a barrier against the harsh, drying environment and keep moisture in the skin where it belongs.

Special Treatments: A fennel seed facial steam once a week will help hydrate the skin and cleanse the pores. Use a moisturizing mask once or twice a week as needed. For both the face and the body, alpha- or beta-hydroxy acid treatments (depending upon your skin's sensitivity) are recommended once a week, as tolerated, to remove dead skin cell build up and promote moisturizer absorption. The nightly use of an emollient eye cream will moisturize the delicate tissue in this area.

Combination Skin

Characteristics: Combination skin results when two skin types occur on one face; there are both dry and oily areas. Generally, the T-zone will appear oily with enlarged pores, visible blackheads, and may be prone to minor breakouts or acne, while the cheeks and neck may feel dry and tight, with possible surface flakiness. Combination skin can be tricky to treat. Most people think that caring for this skin type requires a dual approach, such as using astringent products for the oily areas and moisturizing products for the dry areas. I prefer to use products that regulate and normalize the sebum production for the entire face and throat.

Seasonal Variations: The oily areas tend to normalize a bit in winter while the dry areas get drier. Can be quite aggravating.

Cleansing: A water- or milk-based cleanser used twice a day deep cleans and refines the pores while hydrating and protecting against dryness. Gentle, soap-free products are recommended, especially those containing rosemary, chemotype verbenon, niaouli, everlasting, German chamomile, or spike lavender essential oils.

Toning: To remove excess cleanser, hydrate the skin, and normalize pH, I recommend German chamomile, rose, orange, or lavender floral waters. Four parts yarrow tea mixed with one part vegetable glycerin works wonderfully, too.

Moisturizing: Apply a very light moisturizer all over and apply a bit of nourishing cream to the drier areas if necessary.

Special Treatments: The pores of a combination skin tend to clog easily, thus the dead skin and debris need to be exfoliated on a regular basis. A gentle, pore-refining clay or oatmeal mask followed by an alpha- or beta-hydroxy acid treatment (depending upon your skin's sensitivity) twice a week will be quite beneficial. Once a week, enjoy a lavender and rosemary facial steam to remove impurities from the pores.

Mature Skin

Characteristics: Mature skin usually develops a crepey texture that appears loose and sagging with fine lines and wrinkles. It tends to be dry, but can be normal or oily, and may or may not have age spots, depending on your history of sun exposure.

Seasonal Variations: Winter, with its cold temperatures and dry air, can be a rough season for most mature skins. Flakiness, increased sensitivity, and chapping can occur. Spring and summer are when this skin type thrives, as added humidity means more moisture is available.

Cleansing: For the face, use a gentle, rich lotion or cream cleanser twice a day if you have dry skin or a water-based lotion if your skin is normal-to-oily. Carrot seed essential oil and rosehip seed base oil are highly regenerative and vitalizing and are good additions to your regular cleansing lotion or cream. Make sure to rinse well. For the body, use your favorite cleanser or gentle, natural soap.

Toning: Classic rosewater and glycerin, lavender, or German chamomile floral waters are excellent, gentle toners for facial skin.

Moisturizing: Depending upon the degree of dryness, a nutrient-rich, light- or medium-textured moisturizer that is easily absorbed is important for both the face and the body.

Special Treatments: A honey or moisturizing facial mask, used twice a week, hydrates the skin. An alpha- or beta-hydroxy acid treatment (depending upon your skin's sensitivity) used two to three times a week on both the face and the body will help refine the skin's surface and enhance absorption of your moisturizer. A fennel seed and lavender facial steam once a week will hydrate and cleanse impurities from the pores. As desired, stimulate the circulation and increase blood flow with a facial massage using 2 to 3 drops of carrot seed essential oil mixed with 1 to 2 teaspoons (5–10 ml) of hazelnut oil. If necessary, an eye cream, applied nightly, will ease dryness in this delicate, thin-skinned area.

Sensitive Skin

Characteristics: Do you frequently react to many commonly used skin care products? Does your skin develop rashes, become irritated, blush quickly, overreact to sudden changes in temperature, and sunburn easily? Then it's probably sensitive. Sensitive skin can develop rosacea and couperose conditions (see chapter 13 for a detailed description of couperose complexion).

All skin care products should be fragrance and color free and extremely gentle. Calendula-based products and German chamomile and lavender essential oils may be tolerated well by those of you with sensitive skin.

Seasonal Variations: This skin type tends to be normal-to-dry or very dry and thus winter's crisp, dry air can upset an already irritable complexion. Summer's heat, humidity, and strong sunlight can also wreak havoc, causing sunburn, blemishes, heat rashes, and ruddiness.

Cleansing: Gentle and nonabrasive are the key words here. A chamois facial cloth or a flannel washcloth are ideal to use as a cleansing tool. Avoid terry washcloths, tissues, or loofah pads. For the face, use a water-based lotion or cream cleanser twice a day. For the body, use your favorite cleanser or a gentle, natural soap. Make sure the product you choose does not strip your skin and cause it to feel dry and tight after cleansing.

Toning: Pure aloe vera gel or diluted with equal parts water, classic rose water and glycerin, or German chamomile floral water are generally nonirritating, soothing, and hydrating.

Moisturizing: A rapidly absorbing, light-to-medium weight moisturizer with good hydrating qualities will be most beneficial for this delicate skin on both the face and the body.

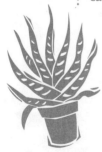

Special Treatments: Antioxidant facial gels, lotions, and creams can help nourish and desensitize this skin type. Keep a German chamomile or lavender floral water spray on hand to prevent dehydration and to soothe irritation. Very low concentrations of alpha- or beta-hydroxy acid can be used, if tolerated, once or twice per week on the face and the body to refine skin texture.

Environmentally Damaged Skin

Characteristics: Deep lines and wrinkles, hyperpigmentation (freckles and age spots), rough texture, and uneven skin tone are telltale signs of the life you've lead if you have this skin type. These characteristics can be the result of sun damage, pollution, climate, excessive living, and just plain neglect. Environmentally damaged skin ages prematurely. It's abused skin and it shows it! It can be oily, normal, or dry.

Seasonal Variations: Each season brings new challenges to environmentally damaged skin. Summer offers the chance for further sun abuse and winter weather makes it feel ultra-parched.

Care: A hydrating, moisturizing sunscreen should be worn every day to prevent further damage to an already abused skin.

Cleansing: For the face, a nonirritating, mild, water-based lotion or cream cleanser fortified with vitamins A, E, and C will deep clean and feed your skin — apply twice daily. A few drops of spike lavender, everlasting, lemongrass, or carrot seed essential oil added to your cleanser will help strengthen the dermal layer and encourage cell renewal. Cleanse your body with your favorite cleanser or gentle, natural soap.

Toning: A gentle, nondrying toner such as lavender floral water will refresh and remove any excess cleanser from the facial skin.

Moisturizing: A lotion or cream enhanced with rosehip seed oil will help to feed, rejuvenate, tone, and support cell membrane functions within the skin of both the face and the body.

Special Treatments: Regular exfoliation all over your body is important to combat the tendency toward flaky skin and uneven skin tone. Use an oatmeal scrub or an alpha- or beta-hydroxy acid treatment (depending upon your skin's sensitivity) twice a week as tolerated to refine skin and cleanse pores. Moisturizing eye creams are a necessity to help prevent this thin area from becoming like dried, crinkled parchment paper.

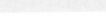

SKINFORMATION

"I've heard it said . . .

by age 20, you have the skin you inherited;
by age 40, you have the skin you deserve; and
by age 60, you have the skin you've earned!

Whether you need to maintain your skin, preserve your skin, or repair your skin, it's never too early and it's never too late to talk to your esthetician about designing a skin care program starting right away."

— From the July 1998 issue of *Smart Skin Care*, published by the American Institute of Esthetics

TOP 10 ENEMIES
FOR ALL SKIN TYPES

1. Smoking. This nasty habit leads to puckering wrinkles around the mouth and fine squinty creases around your eyes. Smoking constricts blood vessels, restricts oxygen uptake, gives a gray color to your complexion, and literally eats up vitamin C, which is necessary for collagen formation.

2. Pollution. The solution to pollution is to avoid it whenever possible. If you live in a dirty, smoggy city and exercise out-of-doors, do so in the early morning when pollution concentration is at its lowest, otherwise, join a gym. Pollution affects your skin in the same way as smoking, minus the puckering and creasing.

3. Dry air. If you work in the typically dry air of a climate-controlled office or live in an arid climate, your skin can easily become parched and thirsty. Keep a hydrating floral water spray handy at all times.

4. Weight loss/gain. Your skin, though quite elastic, is not a rubber band. If you stretch anything too many times, it eventually loses its spring. Stretch marks and sagging, untoned skin can be the result of yo-yo dieting. Try to maintain a relatively constant weight.

5. Excessive pulling on the skin. Makeup and facial products should be applied using a gentle touch. A soft makeup sponge for color application and a light tapping or stroking motion when applying creams and lotions should be employed, otherwise you could encourage sagging.

6. Abusive exfoliation/overzealous cleansing. Washcloths and facial scrubs are designed to exfoliate your skin while cleansing. If you scrub your skin in the same manner used to remove the soap scum from your shower stall, you'll only irritate it and make matters worse, not better.

7. Alcohol. Consumption of alcoholic drinks, no matter how good they may make you feel (temporarily), have absolutely no place in a beautiful skin care regimen. Alcohol dehydrates you from the inside out, taxes your liver, and gobbles up your B vitamins.

8. Drugs. Check with your physician regarding the potential side effects of any medication you are taking. Some drugs may cause photosensitivity (sun sensitivity), dryness, blotchiness, or even mild acne.

9. Constipation. What goes in must exit — regularly! Toxins can build up within your body if your elimination is faulty, but they must eventually escape via some channel. Frequently the path of choice is your skin, so drink plenty of fresh water and eat lots of fiber to keep your plumbing running smoothly (and your skin looking smooth, too).

10. Sunlight. Excessive sun exposure leads to dry, wrinkled, leathery, blotchy, prematurely aged skin and possibly skin cancer. You need your daily dose of vitamin D. Fifteen minutes a day before 10:30 a.m. or after 4:30 p.m., when the sun's rays are not at their most intense, is my recommended daily allotment for sun exposure, without sunscreen. At other times of the day, always wear a sunscreen with an SPF of at least 15 to 25 to help prevent the signs of sun-damaged skin.

FIVE DAILY RITUALS
FOR BEAUTIFUL SKIN

Skin care shouldn't be a complex chore. It should be simple, natural, and basic. And if a few of these straightforward skin care rituals are free for the asking, then so much the better!

I've outlined five of my favorite treatments below. You may be surprised to discover how fundamental these are to achieving glowing skin.

Cleansing Routine

A beauty must! Cleanse your skin twice daily (only once if your skin is dry) using a mild, natural, inexpensive cleanser designed for your skin type. (See chapter 2 for a more in-depth discussion on this topic.)

Cleaning your skin is especially important before going to bed because your body excretes toxins through your skin as you sleep. If facial pores are clogged with makeup and dirt, breakouts can occur. If you perspire a lot in your line of work or you exercise heavily, then rinse off and massage your body with a coarse cloth or loofah before retiring to remove salt and dead skin buildup. Your skin needs to breathe while you sleep!

SKINFORMATION

Sweat is actually good for the skin. It's almost 99 percent water and contains urea and lactic acid, two terrific natural moisturizers that are common ingredients in most moisturizing creams. So go ahead and let 'em see you sweat, it will do your skin a world of good!

Exercise

Try to exercise outside if possible to help oxygenate your cells with fresh air and facilitate waste removal through your skin. If you live in a city, try to find a green space — a park or a greenway — to exercise in. If city streets, with their attendant pollution, are your only outdoor option, exercising in a gym may be a better alternative. Exercises such as walking, biking, rollerblading, and weight lifting improve cardiovascular fitness and muscular endurance, which translates into increased energy and a rosy complexion.

Sleep, Blissful Sleep

Has your "get-up-and-go" got up and gone? Sleep deprivation takes its toll on your face in a hurry. To look and feel your absolute best, you need to get deeply restful, quality sleep. I don't care what else you do to your skin, if you are sleep deprived, your skin will look sallow, dull, tired, and saggy, and with your poor, puffy eyes you will resemble a frog prince or princess. And, of course, your energy level will be less than desirable. Sleep — it's the best-kept skin care secret there is!

Sunlight

Ten to 15 minutes of daily unprotected exposure to sunlight is essential to the health of your bones and your skin. It helps your body absorb calcium due to the skin's ability to convert the sun's rays into vitamin D. Sun exposure helps heal eczema, psoriasis, and acne, and energizes your body. Its warm rays just make you feel good all over.

Always wear a sunscreen with a high SPF if you are going to be exposed for more than fifteen minutes at a time, especially between the hours of 10:30 a.m. and 4:30 p.m. when the sun's rays are at their strongest.

If your dermatologist advises that you avoid the sun entirely, other sources of vitamin D include egg yolks, fish liver oil, vitamin D–supplemented milk or soy milk, organ meats, salmon, sardines, and herring.

Water

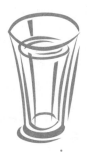

What goes in must go out. Water helps move everything right along. Eight to twelve 8-ounce glasses of pure water a day combined with a fibrous diet will help cleanse your body of toxins and keep your colon functioning as it should. Impurities not disposed of in a timely manner via the internal organs of elimination (such as the kidneys, liver, lungs, and large intestine), will find an alternate exit, namely your skin, which is sometimes referred to as the "third kidney." Pimples and rashes may develop as your body tries to unload its wastes through your skin. Water also keeps your skin hydrated and moisturized, so drink up!

SKINFORMATION

Skin disorders such as eczema, psoriasis, acne, hives, excess perspiration, and a pale complexion can be triggered or worsened by stress. Techniques for reducing stress include: exercise, ample sleep, facial and body massage, reflexology, deep breathing, biofeedback, reiki, time with close friends and family, and recreation.

PROFESSIONAL TIPS
TO KEEP YOUR SKIN IN SUPER SHAPE

◆ Try to have a professional facial at least twice a year.
◆ Keep a mister bottle of either purified water or aromatic hydrosol handy at all times to refresh and hydrate your skin whenever you start to feel dry. This is especially important if you're a frequent flyer.
◆ Drink, drink, drink . . . at least eight glasses of purified water every day.
◆ Use sunscreen daily.
◆ Cleanse, tone, and moisturize twice a day with products specifically created for your skin type. As you get older, reevaluate your skin type. Everything changes with age!
◆ Eat a healthy diet and get plenty of exercise.
◆ Learn to manage the stress in your life. Stress wreaks havoc on even the most beautiful skin.

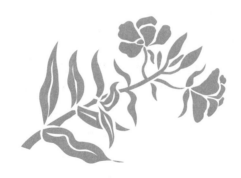

CHAPTER 13
Natural Solutions for Common Skin Problems

It's time to face your complexion challenges armed with knowledge. Because your skin is a living, complex system of intertwining processes, your focus needs to shift from merely addressing symptoms to actually supporting the healthy functioning of your skin. Attune your skin. Let it reflect a harmonious balance between the internal workings of your body and the exposure it receives from its external environment.

Whether your quest is to postpone the inevitability of aging, cure your cystic acne, lighten your age spots, educate yourself about skin cancer prevention, or quench your dry skin's thirst, you've come to the right spot. Dermatological medications and topical chemical treatments are occasionally necessary to help manage troublesome skin afflictions, but these drugs can have irritating and even potentially irreversible side effects and should be avoided whenever possible. I feel that 90 percent of the time there is a natural solution to every health problem that crosses your path. Common skin maladies are not an exception.

Remember, achieving flawless skin is not an instantaneous process. Nature takes time to work her magic. Your skin didn't assume its present condition overnight, so have patience. In time, your skin will reveal the true beauty within you.

A good, holistically orientated dermatologist can help guide you through the maze of toxic treatments and design a beneficial treatment plan you can live with. An esthetician trained in holistic skin care can be of assistance in designing a skin care program to augment your dermatologist's recommendations and can also show you how to properly care for your skin at home.

The advice of your dermatologist and esthetician can prove invaluable when it comes to matters of the skin, but remember — only you can take control of your appearance and health. The more you strive to live in harmony with your surroundings, eat a nutritious diet, and take proper care of your skin, the more benefits your skin will reap. So, read on and take charge of your skin's health. Only you can change the outlook of the skin you're in!

WHAT'S THE DIFFERENCE?

A **dermatologist** is a medical doctor specializing in disorders of the skin. A dermatologist can prescribe drugs and perform surgical procedures.

An **esthetician** is someone who has completed a specified amount of training in esthetics required by his or her state (usually between 300 and 600 hours). An esthetician usually has training in specialties such as makeup artistry, aromatherapy, nutrition, massage, reflexology, manual lymph drainage, waxing, and pre- and postoperative skin care.

ACNE

Acne vulgaris, or acne, as it is commonly known, is the most common skin disease. Acneic skin is oily, shiny, and blemished and has enlarged pores (which are often clogged) and blackheads and whiteheads covering its surface. Acne manifests on the face and frequently on the neck, chest, shoulders, and back. Pimples can be red and inflamed and, if not properly addressed, can lead to larger pimples (pustules) and deeper lumps (cysts or nodules). More often than not, a person who suffers from acne will have oily hair as well, which exacerbates the problem by causing breakouts around the hairline.

Causes of Acne

According to dermatologists, acne is caused by the hormone testosterone, which stimulates production of oil (sebum), which promotes acne. It is not caused by poor hygiene, but it

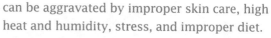

can be aggravated by improper skin care, high heat and humidity, stress, and improper diet.

Acne begins when a sebaceous follicle is obstructed by a combination of cellular debris and sebum. This obstruction forms a *comedone,* or plug, commonly referred to as either a blackhead (if it has a brown or black head) or a whitehead or milia (if it has a white head). If a whitehead ruptures beneath the surface of the skin, either involuntarily or because it was squeezed or improperly extracted, a chain reaction is triggered. First a pimple forms, which becomes inflamed as bacteria begin to grow in the surrounding tissue. Now this simple pimple has become a pustule and looks red and angry, filled with yellow pus. If the situation worsens and the infection moves deeper, a painful, inflamed nodule could form, which looks like an ugly, round knot on the skin. Should the nodule progress, a sac filled with fluid forms, called a cyst. Cysts are deep, serious lesions that require medical treatment.

There are four grades of acne:

Grade I: In mild cases of acne vulgaris, the skin displays a few minor pimples, whiteheads, and blackheads.

Grade II: The skin has more pimples and/or pustules (a pimple containing pus), and pores are more frequently clogged.

Grade III: The skin displays a greater inflammation of lesions in the form of pustules (large and small) and a further increase in blackhead and whitehead development.

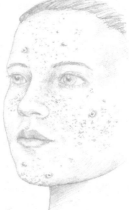

In the Grade II level of acne, whiteheads, blackheads, and pustules are obvious.

Grade IV: Many large pustules, nodules (deep pustules), and cysts are often accompanied by areas heavily congested with blackheads and whiteheads. This grade of acne should be treated only by a dermatologist.

Acne is not just for adolescents. True, acne commonly rears its ugly head with the hormonal surge of the preteen years, but many cases occur in adults, especially women. Adult-onset acne tends to be due to increased stress, overzealous cleansing, and the hormonal changes of pregnancy, menstrual cycles, menopause, or as a result of hormonal abnormalities, including the increased testosterone productivity that may accompany ovarian cysts. Unlike teenage acne, adult acne usually confines itself to the chin and jawline areas, though I've also seen it flare up on the nose and cheeks.

Although both men and women respond to stress with a rise in adrenal hormones, women, in particular, respond by overproducing testosterone, thereby causing adult-onset acne. Just how does increased stress induce acne? According to Robert and Webster Stone, authors of *Zit Wars: The Battle for Great Skin,* stress activates the hypothalamus, which stimulates the pituitary gland, thus stimulating the adrenal glands, which then release testosterone, stimulating the oil glands to produce oil (sebum), which promotes acne.

HANDS OFF!

Remember as a teen when your mother told you not to pick at your blemishes because it could make them worse? Well, she was right! Self-treatment of acne, including picking or squeezing with fingernails, needles, or metal implements is not helpful. It can cause your simple pimple to rupture under the surface of the skin, become inflamed, and lead to either a permanent pitted scar or possibly an ugly, painful cyst. There is a correct way to "pop" your pimples — see pages 258–259.

Prevention

Here is a bit of sage advice toward the prevention of this annoying skin disease:

Identify your skin type. Take care of your skin, treat it well, and it will bless you with years of beauty. Neglect it, and it can be the bane of your existence. See a skin professional and find out what type of skin you have and how to properly take care of its needs, then follow their recommendations to the letter.

Choose cosmetics wisely. Ideally, facial makeup, lotions, and creams should be hypoallergenic, noncomedogenic, and nonacnegenic; these products are unlikely to cause allergies and won't clog your pores. *Acne cosmetica* is the term for cosmetic-induced acne and is quite common.

Supplement your diet. Some supplements, such as vitamin A, zinc, cod liver oil, borage oil, and evening primrose oil, have been shown to be helpful in many cases of acne, from mild to severe. Cod liver oil and evening primrose oil have indeed been a blessing to my mild case of adult-onset acne. I take one tablespoon of cod liver oil every other day and one 1,300 mg capsule of evening primrose oil daily.

Be gentle to your skin. Avoid overzealous cleansing of your skin as well as industrial strength facial scrubs. In an attempt to rid themselves of pimples and blackheads — which, incidentally, can't be washed away — many sufferers scrub their faces with either a washcloth and soap or an exfoliant product, several times a day, like it was the kitchen floor. This acts only to dry the skin's surface and stimulate more oil production beneath. Use a gentle hand and soothing, mild products specifically designed for your skin type when cleansing.

Practice stress reduction. I can't emphasize this enough! If you're an adult woman suffering with adult-onset acne, I can almost guarantee that your disturbing skin condition will subside if you lower the stress in your life. Yoga, reiki, reflexology, walking, running, rollerblading, meditation, gardening . . . whatever it takes for you to relax, partake of it frequently. The less stress in your life, the less adrenaline and testosterone your body will produce.

Beware of iodine intake. A few sensitive individuals experience irritation of the follicles when excess iodides in the diet are excreted through the sebaceous ducts. To determine if iodine is aggravating your acne, minimize or avoid foods containing iodides, such as kelp, liver, fish and shellfish, corn, white onions, asparagus, milk, and beef. Certain supplements contain high levels of iodine too, so check the label. Additionally, some brands of birth control pills contain iodides — ask your doctor if your brand contains iodides, and if so, ask for a different prescription.

Hydrate. Drink plenty of pure water to flush out toxins and keep the skin hydrated.

Sleep well. If you "party hearty" too often, it will show up on your skin. Eight hours of sleep each night (or whatever it takes to make you feel rested and lively) is imperative.

Avoid stimulants. Stay away from or limit stimulants such as caffeine and cigarettes. They sap valuable nutrients that are essential for skin health, such as vitamins B and C, from your system.

Don't touch. Keep your hands off your face. If you have oily hair, shampoo daily and keep your hair in a style that is up and off your face.

Treatments for Acne

To heal or at least lessen the severity of your acne, you must normalize or attempt to reduce the sebum production in your skin. This can be accomplished in several ways. Drug therapy could include topical treatments such as benzoyl peroxide; salicylic-acid lotions, creams, and toners; tretinoin; sodium sulfacetamide lotion; or Retin-A. Accutane, an oral medication, is very popular and extremely effective, but can have terrible side effects and its use must be monitored by a dermatologist. If your acne is severe, other oral antibiotics such as tetracycline, minocycline, or erythromycin might be prescribed. Though these therapies can be successful by reducing bacteria and comedone formation, they can have unfortunate side effects that range from facial and oral dryness and chapped lips to birth defects in pregnant women.

Alternatively, you could choose a more natural, holistically supportive approach to treating your complexion, sans side effects. There are many gentle yet effective herbal tonics and natural cleansers that can be used to encourage more harmonious functioning of your skin.

Regardless of which route you choose, your acne will not heal overnight. Dermatologists say to allow at least 1 to 6 months for your problem skin to show signs of improvement. In order to head off future acne eruptions, you must adhere to a strict regimen of home and professional care. Make a commitment to stick with your treatments. Consistency is the key to clearer skin.

FACE IT

This herbal tea, formulated by Jean Argus of Jean's Greens (see Resources), is a tasty way to nourish your body and aid in liver detoxification. It comes from an old Mexican formula and is used daily to improve skin. It's available in bulk from her mail-order catalog. I highly recommend it.

4 tablespoons (60 ml) dried oatstraw

4 tablespoons (60 ml) dried figwort

2 tablespoons (30 ml) dried sarsaparilla

2 tablespoons (30 ml) dried burdock

1½ teaspoons (7.5 ml) dried yellow dock

½ teaspoon (2.5 ml) dried licorice root

1 teaspoon (5 ml) dried stevia (to sweeten)

Yield: Enough for approximately 30–35 cups (7.5–9 l) of tea.

To make:
1. Mix the herbs together.
2. To 4 cups (1 liter) of boiling water, add 4–6 heaping teaspoons (20–30 ml) of the herb mixture and immediately remove from heat.
3. Cover and steep for 10–15 minutes.
4. Strain and cool if desired.

To use:
Consume 4 cups (1 liter) daily as an internal skin tonic. For maximum benefit, continue regular consumption over 4–6 months to see desired results.

Liver tonics. The liver is primarily responsible for keeping hormones such as testosterone in check. Most herbalists, if asked to recommend a formula for clearing the skin of chronic skin problems such as eczema, psoriasis, rashes, or acne, will usually include herbs to improve the functioning of the liver, such as those in the Face It tea formula (see page 250).

Natural cleansers. Acneic skin should be kept scrupulously clean and the follicles regularly deep cleansed and kept that way to prevent future breakouts. The cleansing products you choose should be water-based and free of perfumes, dyes, and most chemicals. Your aim is to thoroughly clean but not strip your skin's protective acid barrier. Always rinse with tepid (not hot) water, followed by an herbal toner (such as my Yarrow Skin Toner) and an oil-free moisturizer or aromatic hydrosol spray to prevent dehydration.

YARROW SKIN TONER

This astringent liquid will serve as an effective herbal antiseptic to kill the bacteria that accompanies acne development, help balance the production of excess sebum, and reduce the visible oil on your face. I recommend it for normal, oily, or acneic complexions.

2 cups (500 ml) boiling water

2 heaping teaspoons (10 ml) dried yarrow or 4 heaping teaspoons (20 ml) fresh

10 drops tea tree essential oil

5 drops inula graveolens or eucalyptus essential oil

Yield: 2 cups (500 ml)

To make:

1. Add yarrow to boiling water, remove from heat, cover and steep for 30 minutes until nice and strong.

2. Strain and cool. Add essential oils.

3. Store in a jar or squeeze bottle in the refrigerator for up to 1 month.

To use:

May be applied using a cotton square as a toner to your entire face or body after cleansing, or whenever you need degreasing. Feels especially good if chilled and splashed on post-workouts.

Regular exfoliation through the use of alpha- or beta-hydroxy acid products or clay-based masks is of utmost importance to help reduce breakouts and remove dead skin buildup that could clog pores. Use one of my gentle exfoliation recipes or find a mild natural product that includes soothing ingredients such as German chamomile, lavender, comfrey, and calendula.

Sebum maintenance. I live in a coastal community on Cape Cod, Massachusetts, and when the summer heat and humidity strike in July and August, my normal-to-dry skin does an about-face and pumps out the oil. For 2 months I alter my cleansing routine to remove the excess oil and shine. I rely on gentle soaps from my natural products company, September's Sun Herbal Soap & Skin Care (see Resources), that are very gentle and don't strip my skin of all its protective oils. After a cleansing with natural soap, I apply an herbal toner and follow up with the Sebum Balancing Formula, which helps to reduce and balance the oil production in my skin.

SEBUM BALANCING FORMULA

2 tablespoons (30 ml) almond or hazelnut oil

4 drops spike lavender essential oil

4 drops eucalyptus essential oil

3 drops blue cypress essential oil

2 drops lemongrass essential oil (optional)

Yield: 1 ounce (30 ml)

To make: Combine all ingredients in a small, 1-ounce (30-ml) glass bottle, and cap tightly. Store formula in a refrigerator for up to 1 year.

To use:

1. Apply on clean, damp skin after using an aromatic hydrosol or toner.

2. Place 2–4 drops in the palm of your hand and add a few drops of water.

3. Rub palms together to warm and mix the liquids and then press gently onto your face and neck. Don't rub or massage your face too aggressively. Your skin should rapidly absorb this formula.

Treating Blackhead Outbreaks

Blackheads can develop singularly or in clusters anywhere the skin is particularly oily, especially the face, neck, shoulders, chest, and back. At times they appear flush with the skin's surface and are barely detectable and other times are slightly raised, very black, and obvious. If infected, a blackhead may be surrounded by pus.

Blackheads are formed by obstructions in your pores, or hair follicles. Oil-producing sebaceous glands, which are connected to your hair follicles, secrete a mixture of fats, proteins, cholesterol, and inorganic salts onto the surface of your skin to keep it supple, hold in moisture, and keep your hair pliable and shiny. When your pores (follicles) become filled with solidified sebum, bacteria, and keratinized skin cells, the oil plug moves upward and outward, dilating the opening of the pore and making it quite visible. The blackness is not caused by dirt; rather, a combination of skin pigment cells and exposure to oxygen gives the oil plug its color. A whitehead, on the other hand, has a layer of skin covering it and has not been exposed to oxygen; it remains white.

To prevent the formation of these unsightly black oil plugs and enlarged pores, your skin must be kept deep-down clean. Cleanse twice daily with an oil-free cleanser, then apply an herbal toner for oily skin (such as strong peppermint or sage tea) or an aromatic hydrosol. Follow up with an oil-free moisturizer if necessary. An oil-absorbing clay mask, such as the Fruit Paste Mask (see page 254), should be used in blackhead prone areas once or twice a week to absorb excess oil and exfoliate dead skin cells.

QUICK BLACKHEAD CLEANSER

To prevent blackheads, try this quick formula for a cleanser: 1 teaspoon (5 ml) liquid castile soap (available in most health food stores) mixed with 1 drop tea tree or thyme essential oil. You can mix it right at the sink as you're washing up.

FRUIT PASTE MASK

A simple yet effective treatment for blackhead outbreaks.

1 tablespoon (15 ml)
white cosmetic clay
2 teaspoons (10 ml)
freshly squeezed
apple, pineapple, or
grape juice

Yield: 1 treatment

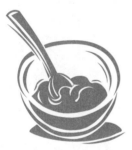

To make: Combine ingredients in a small bowl and stir until a smooth, spreadable paste forms. If the paste is too thick, add more juice; if too runny, add a bit more clay.

To use:

1. Spread a thick paste over freshly cleansed, blackhead prone area(s) and allow to dry completely, about 20 minutes.

2. Rinse with cool or tepid water. Pat dry and apply a dab of oil-free moisturizer mixed with a drop of tea tree or eucalyptus essential oil to the area. May be used once or twice weekly or as needed to keep pores clean and clear.

Blackhead Extraction Procedure

Blackheads can be removed by extraction. When the oil plug is removed the pore will appear smaller, but since the pore has been enlarged and filled with a blackhead, chances are it will become filled again in a few weeks unless you are extra diligent about your skin care regimen. You'll need:

- ◆ Two squares of flannel cloth, large enough to comfortably wrap around your index fingers
- ◆ A washcloth
- ◆ A bowl holding 4 to 5 cups (1,000 to 1,250 ml) of very warm water or chamomile tea
- ◆ Two tablespoons (30 ml) Epsom salts or sea salt

Step 1: Cleanse the skin thoroughly with a gentle, oil-free cleanser.

Step 2: Stir the salt into the warm water or tea and stir until dissolved.

Step 3: Soak the washcloth in the salty water and squeeze out the excess liquid. Place washcloth over blackhead(s) you wish to extract and hold it there for about 5 minutes to soften the skin and sebum and ready the skin for extraction. Concentrate on one area of your face or body at a time.

Step 4: When ready, dampen the flannel squares in the same liquid as you did the washcloth and then wrap them around your index fingers. While holding the skin taut between your two fingers, begin a very gentle squeezing and lifting motion on either side of the blackhead. Do not apply too much pressure. You should see a semi-solid white or yellow waxy secretion exude from the pore opening. If you don't, then the blackhead is not ready to come out and if you proceed, you'll only damage the surrounding tissue and possibly cause a nasty pimple. Continue this procedure on other blackheads.

Step 5: Following the extraction, use the Fruit Paste Mask (see page 254) on the treated areas to remove even more sebum, minimize pore size, and reduce possible inflammation. Add a drop of German chamomile or everlasting essential oil to the recipe, as these ingredients have powerful anti-inflammatory properties.

Treating Pimple Outbreaks

Everyone is well aware of what a pesky pimple looks like. That red, slightly raised spot that may or may not be infected with a creamy yellow center (pus) seems to always appear at just the wrong time and in the wrong place. I'm not discussing full-fledged acne here, just a minor pimple outbreak and how to deal with it.

When a pore or hair follicle becomes clogged by excess dead skin cells, sebum, and bacteria and ruptures beneath the skin, a pimple forms. A breakout can be triggered by stress, hormone fluctuation, improper cleansing, and overactive sebaceous glands. You don't have to have particularly oily skin to have a pimple, or two or three. I sometimes break out during the winter when my skin tends to be dehydrated. Everyone gets a pimple from time to time; no one is completely immune.

Quick tips. Here are some valuable points to consider to help prevent the occasional pimple. You may recognize some of the advice, as it was given earlier for treating acne, and indeed you'll find the same advice repeated throughout this chapter. The point? Even if you have relatively healthy, problem-free skin, you still need to follow good skin care basics in order to maintain a vibrant complexion.

◆ Keep your hands off your face.
◆ Stick to a proper cleansing regimen for your skin type.
◆ If you spend lots of time on the telephone, sanitize it daily and apply an astringent toner to your lower cheek, jawline, and neck.
◆ Avoid restrictive clothing if possible, or at least apply a bit of medicated cornstarch or arrowroot powder to absorb perspiration and keep the area dry and relatively friction-free.
◆ Grow out your bangs and get them off your face, or keep your hair scrupulously clean and oil free.
◆ Get rid of the stress in your life or at least minimize it.
◆ Get plenty of exercise and fresh air, and eat a healthy diet.
◆ Drink plenty of water to flush toxins from your system and keep your skin hydrated.

Tea tree oil. According to an article in the August 1998 issue of *Vegetarian Times* by Norine Dworkin, "Tea tree oil is known as an effective acne fighter. A 1990 study by Lederle Laboratories and Royal Prince Alfred Hospital in Great Britain found that a 5 percent tea tree oil gel was as effective as benzoyl peroxide in treating acne, with less drying, stinging, and redness. Use a commercially prepared ointment, available in natural health stores, or dab undiluted oil right on pimples."

Yes, tea tree essential oil is a wonderful spot treatment. Its antiseptic and antibacterial properties make it a superior choice for fighting pimples whenever they arise.

PIMPLE MAGIC JUICE

This essential oil formula really seems to help heal breakouts in a hurry!

2 tablespoons (30 ml) store-bought aloe vera juice
2 drops thyme essential oil (chemotype linalol)
2 drops tea tree essential oil
2 drops spike lavender essential oil
2 drops eucalyptus essential oil

Yield: 1 ounce (30 ml)

To make: Combine all ingredients in a 1-ounce (30-ml) bottle and shake well. Store in a cool, dry, dark place for up to 4 months, or refrigerate for up to 1 year. **To use:** Dab directly on pimple after cleansing. May use up to 3 times daily. If irritation occurs, reduce usage.

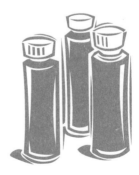

Pimple Extraction Procedure

To effectively "pop" a pimple, it must first come to a very visible head with the pus showing prominently in the center. A layer of crust may have formed over the top. Do not attempt to extract any pimples that do not have this appearance or you could cause scarring or the formation of a cyst. You'll need:

◆ Two squares of flannel cloth, large enough to comfortably wrap around your index fingers
◆ A washcloth
◆ A sewing needle
◆ A bowl holding 4 to 5 cups (1,000 to 1,250 ml) of very warm water or pepperment tea
◆ 4 drops thyme essential oil
◆ 2 drops German chamomile essential oil
◆ 2 tablespoons (30 ml) Epsom salts or sea salt
◆ Matches or rubbing alcohol

Step 1: Cleanse the area thoroughly.

Step 2: Add the essential oils and salt to the warm water or tea. Stir until the salt is dissolved.

Step 3: Soak the washcloth in the salty water and squeeze out the excess liquid. Hold the cloth over the pimple for a few minutes to soften the sebum, which will make extraction easier.

Step 4: Sterilize a needle in a match flame or rubbing alcohol. Use it to prick the center surface skin of the pimple carefully, to open the top layer of epidermis. This ensures that the pus will break through on the surface of the skin and not be pushed into the lower layers, where it could cause further inflammation.

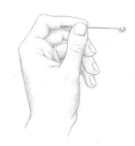

Be careful to prick just the top layer of skin over the pimple.

Step 5: When ready, dampen the flannel squares in the same liquid as you did the washcloth and then wrap them around your index fingers. (Do not use your fingernails, as they can cause scars.) Apply gentle pressure on each side of the pimple with a lifting, slightly squeezing motion. The debris should ooze from the clogged pore. If it doesn't, try twice more on different sides of the pimple, then stop. You don't want to cause deeper damage. Blood or clear fluid should ooze from the pore following the pus extraction.

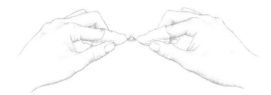

Gently apply a lifting, slightly squeezing pressure to force the debris up and out from the clogged pore.

Step 6: Apply Pimple Magic Juice (see page 257) or a dab of tea tree essential oil to the area to cleanse and disinfect.

Consulting the Experts

See an Esthetician If: An esthetician can be of great assistance in the care of acneic skin. She can provide a gentle facial or back treatment and steam or hot packs to soften the skin and loosen hardened sebum. Depending on the severity of your condition, she may suggest a series of deep-pore cleansings to thoroughly remove the pore-clogging debris, and will often work in conjunction with any prescribed dermatological treatments. Additionally, she can educate you as to which home treatment products are most beneficial for your particular skin condition.

See a Dermatologist If: Some skin conditions, such as severe cystic or nodular acne, require the care of a doctor. If your acne is unresponsive to home treatments and visits to an esthetician are not producing the desired results, consult a dermatologist. Locate a doctor who is holistically oriented, one who will treat your whole person — mind, body, and spirit — and not just the symptomatic spots on your face.

PREVENTING SKIN CANCER

Your chances of getting skin cancer can be greatly reduced if you follow these tips (from the American Academy of Dermatology):

♦ Try to avoid the sun between 10:30 a.m. and 4:30 p.m., when the sun's rays are the strongest.
♦ Apply a broad-spectrum sunscreen with a sun protection factor (SPF) of at least 15.
♦ Reapply sunscreen every 2 hours when outdoors, even on cloudy days.
♦ Wear protective, tightly woven clothing, such as a long-sleeved shirt and pants.
♦ Wear a 4-inch (10-cm) wide-brimmed hat and sunglasses, even when walking short distances.
♦ Stay in the shade whenever possible.
♦ Avoid reflective surfaces, which can reflect up to 85 percent of the sun's damaging rays.
♦ Protect children by keeping them out of the sun, minimizing sun exposure and applying sunscreens beginning at 6 months of age.
♦ If you notice a change in the size, shape, or appearance of a mole, see a dermatologist.

CELLULITE

Cellulite is the dimpled, lumpy skin that most often appears on the thighs, hips, buttocks, and stomach. Cellulite is not a type of fat, but rather is a result of the relationship between skin and the fat layer beneath it. It affects women more than men because women tend to have more subcutaneous fat and slightly thinner skin.

Causes

If you were to ask ten different skin care and body-care experts, ranging from dermatologists to estheticians to massage therapists, to state the causes of cellulite, you'd get ten different answers. Here are some of the answers I received:

◆ There's no such thing as cellulite. It's just plain old fat. The cause is simply a lack of exercise and overeating.
◆ It's a result of stagnant circulation in various areas between the torso and the knees.
◆ Cellulite is a type of fat that traps extra water beneath the skin's surface, causing a puckered appearance.
◆ Cellulite is caused by toxins in the diet, such as artificial sweeteners, preservatives, and additives, which the body stores in fat cells.
◆ The appearance of cellulite is more apparent when the underlying muscle is untoned and flabby. In an athletic body the visible dimpling of the fat layer, if evident at all, is minimal.
◆ Cellulite is one of the side effects of a constipated colon and insufficient water intake, resulting in an overaccumulation of toxins. When toxins are not being released through the proper channels — the skin, kidneys, liver, and colon — they are stored in the fat tissue, isolated from the body and out of harm's way.
◆ Cellulite is a combination of fat, water, and wastes trapped beneath the skin in pockets within the connective fiber bands that hold the skin in place. As the amount of these materials increases, the pockets bulge, causing the familiar cottage-cheese effect.

All of these "causes" of cellulite ring true to a certain degree. Cellulite does consist of fatty tissue, water, and toxins, and the degree to which it affects you depends upon the types of food you consume as well as the amount and type of exercise you get. Although it can be difficult to eradicate, there are ways to eliminate it or at least minimize its appearance.

Preventing Cellulite Development

If you're one of the few people who isn't afflicted with cellulite, you're either very young or very fortunate. Even female athletes who work out more than 2 hours a day can still have a minor amount of cellulite on their thighs and buttocks. However, there are several lifestyle "adjustments" you can make — if they're not already a part of your routine — that will not only keep you healthier in general but will also help prevent the formation of, or further development of, cellulite.

◆ Get up, move, and sweat! Daily, vigorous aerobic exercise is paramount, so fight your sedentary tendencies. Try jogging, walking, dancing, bicycling, or rollerblading to stimulate circulation throughout your body, especially from the waist down (the area most commonly affected by cellulite).
◆ Begin a regular weight-lifting routine to keep your underlying muscles toned and tight.
◆ Drink, drink, drink — water, that is. An ample intake of water will keep toxins flowing right out of your body.
◆ Eat a proper, balanced diet with as many whole, unrefined foods as possible.
◆ Avoid salty foods like the plague! Salt causes your body to retain water, which can exacerbate the appearance of cellulite.
◆ Stop smoking. Smoking impairs circulation and adds poisonous toxins to your bloodstream.
◆ Keep alcohol and caffeine consumption to a minimum. They contribute more toxins for your body to deal with, and they sap your body of valuable nutrients essential for skin health.
◆ Stay within your normal, healthy weight range. Cellulite is more pronounced if you are overweight.

Treatments for Cellulite

All professionals who treat cellulite agree upon one thing: Cellulite is a chronic condition that requires continual treatment and maintenance. It is not a condition that you pay attention to one day and not the next. As soon as you stop preventive or treatment measures, cellulite will begin to build up again. To properly treat cellulite, you must make whatever method you decide upon a part of your regular routine.

The following treatment suggestions consist of diet and exercise programs. They really work for those who are motivated and diligent. You must be consistent in your efforts for smooth, tight, firm skin to prevail. Cellulite will respond positively to your new lifestyle habits, but it may be a long process. Remember, you didn't get into the shape you're in overnight — fat and cellulite will take just as long to disappear.

Please note, if you are overweight, I recommend a visit to your physician to alert her or him of your intention to begin a new diet and exercise program.

Aerobic weight lifting. This type of exercise combines the cardiovascular benefits of aerobics with strengthening and muscle-building weights. It makes you really sweat and seems to carve the fat right off my thighs and buttocks as fast as a hot knife through butter. When I'm consistent with this type of exercise, I usually see results in as little as 10 days. Unfortunately, very few workout tapes offer this type of exercise combination. Call your local gym to see if they offer classes.

Yoga. If you've never taken a yoga-for-strength class, you may think that yoga is for people who can't do strenuous exercise. That assumption couldn't be further from the truth. The practice of yoga consists of performing a series of postures that strengthen your muscles and joints using your own body weight for resistance. When you hold a pose, you're working your muscles isometrically (without moving). I find that yoga tones and elongates my muscles, making for a leaner, more lithe look. It builds balance, coordination, and strength, and is wonderfully de-stressing as well.

Dry brushing. This is a wonderful technique for improving skin tone, circulation, and lymph flow, and for shedding dry skin. See pages 6–7 for how-to instructions.

Diet. Reduce your consumption of refined and simple carbohydrates, including white flour, sugar and sugar substitutes, chips, cake, cookies, crackers, popcorn, and french fries, to name a few. Such starchy, sugary foods offer minimal nutritional value, and if eaten in excess, cause weight gain and water retention.

ANTI-CELLULITE BATH TREATMENT

The rosemary and lavender essential oils in this formula pamper and condition your skin, while the juniper and cypress essential oils exert a diuretic action, helping to reduce water retention. The salt aids in toxin elimination and muscle relaxation.

2 teaspoons (10 ml) almond, avocado, or sesame oil
1 teaspoon (5 ml) honey
1 teaspoon (5 ml) vodka, gin, or rum
2 drops juniper essential oil
3 drops cypress essential oil
4 drops lavender angustifolia essential oil
3 drops rosemary (chemotype linalol) essential oil
½ cup (125 ml) Epsom salts

Yield: 1 bath treatment

To prepare the bath:
1. Blend the oil, honey, alcohol, and essential oils in a small bowl. Set aside.
2. Start the water running in the tub and add the salts; stir them around until they are dissolved.
3. When the tub is full, pour in the oily mixture.
To use:
Soak for approximately 20 minutes. Massage the cellulite-afflicted areas while you are soaking to help break down the fatty deposits. Then get out and briskly dry your skin using a thickly napped towel. Follow up with an application of body lotion to which you have added a drop of each of the essential oils in the ingredients list. You may partake of this bath up to 3 times a week.

Consulting the Experts

See an Esthetician If: If you want to temporarily reduce the appearance of cellulite, your esthetician can help. She may offer an herbal body wrap treatment, which stimulates circulation, helps eliminate toxins and excess water, and revitalizes the skin's texture and tone. This is also a super way to relax. However, keep in mind that the small amount of weight shed, the tightening of the skin, and/or the inches lost are the result of water loss and will return within a day or two.

Estheticians who are trained in deep tissue massage may offer a series of anticellulite treatments. This requires that you receive an aggressive 1 hour massage (usually a lower body massage) 1 or 2 times a week, depending upon the severity of your condition, for a total of approximately 18 treatments. The benefits include improved circulation and lymph flow, reduction of lactic acid, relaxed muscles, and improved skin texture. Following a massage, you may notice an increased need to urinate, as fluid has been pushed out of the subcutaneous tissues and must be eliminated. This fluid loss will result in a slight reduction in measurement. Maintenance services are required at the rate of one or two treatments a month thereafter. (Unfortunately, this can be quite time consuming and expensive.) Please note, if you have a heart condition, varicose veins, or diabetes, you should avoid this type of procedure.

See a Dermatologist If: If all your diligent effort in trying to reduce the amount of cellulite on your body has failed, your dermatologist may be of some assistance. A dermatologist can perform liposuction, a procedure in which a small suctioning device is inserted under the skin to remove fat cells. As wonderful and easy as it sounds, though, liposuction can be painful and expensive, and it may even worsen the dimpling and puckering symptoms in some patients. Not everyone is a good candidate for this type of surgery. Talk it over thoroughly with your doctor and discuss the pros and cons before deciding to undergo this surgical technique.

CHAPPED, DRY LIPS

You know what chapped lips feel like — dry, tight, flaky, cracked, and burning. All you want to do is lick them and put out the fire. Chapped lips are red or purplish in color and seem to absorb any moisture that you put on them and then scream for more.

Causes of Chapped Lips

Your lips, unlike the rest of your skin, do not contain any sebaceous or sweat glands and therefore cannot moisturize themselves; they constantly need re-wetting. Normally, the small amount of saliva that reaches the surface of your lips via the tip of your tongue is sufficient to keep them moist. However, if the lip tissue is damaged from heat, cold, lipsticks, dry air, smoking, sunburn, herpes, infection, or topical or oral medications, your saliva will not be sufficient to prevent your lips from becoming dehydrated.

Prevention

Follow these tips to keep your smoocher soft and kissable:

- When venturing out into the sun, be it the beach or bright ski slope, don't forget to apply a lip balm with an SPF of 15 or higher. Lips can get sunburned, too!
- Brush your lips! After brushing your teeth, gently brush your lips as well. "Not only does it take away any chapping, but it plumps up the lip temporarily for that sought-after 'pouty' look," says Diane Irons, author of *The World's Best-Kept Beauty Secrets*.
- Apply a lip balm frequently throughout the day to create a moisture resistant barrier on your lips that will help prevent moisture loss.
- Keep hydrated! Drink lots of water throughout the day.
- Dab honey on your lips to soothe and protect. Honey acts as a humectant — it draws moisture from the air to your skin, thus keeping your lips soft and plump.
- Castor oil, the first ingredient in most lipsticks, can be applied straight out of the bottle for a glossy look.

Treatments for Chapped Lips

Chapped or chronically dry lips need constant moisture and protection from the elements. So pamper your lips with my delicious lip balm formula.

LIP SLICKER

5 tablespoons (75 ml) castor or jojoba oil (use 6 tablespoons [90 ml] if you prefer a thinner, glossier texture)

1 tablespoon (15 ml) beeswax

1 teaspoon (5 ml) chopped alkanet root for deep red color (optional)

1 teaspoon (5 ml) honey or vegetable glycerine

10 drops peppermint, orange, or lemongrass essential oil for flavor (**or** add 10 drops carrot seed essential oil to revitalize dry, chapped lip skin **or** 10 drops of either tea tree or eucalyptus essential oil to treat cold sores and cracked, bleeding lips)

Yield: Approximately 3 ounces (90 ml)

To make:

1. Combine the oil and beeswax in a small saucepan over low heat or in a double boiler and warm until the wax is melted. Remove from heat.

2. If you desire a colorant, add alkanet root now and let steep for 1 hour. Remelt oil and wax until liquid, strain out alkanet, and proceed with the recipe.

3. While oil and wax mixture is still a warm liquid, add honey and essential oil(s), and blend the mixture thoroughly. Pour into ¼–½ ounce (7–15 g) tins or cosmetic jars while still hot. Will keep for up to 1 year if refrigerated.

To use: Since a lip balm adds no moisture to your lips, it is recommended that you provide moisture first. Apply a drop of water or a dab of honey to the lip surface and lightly pat with a tissue to remove the excess. Then slather on a good layer of sweet or medicated lip balm to seal in the moisture you just applied.

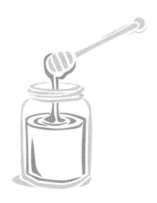

Consulting the Experts

See an Esthetician If: If you don't want to make your own lip-healing formula, your skin care professional will carry a tube or two of lip balm containing beeswax, castor oil, and/or vitamin E in her salon, though for the price, you can't beat making your own!

See a Dermatologist If: A common side effect of topical or oral prescription drugs, especially acne medications, is dry, tight, burning lips. If this occurs and the above recommendations don't provide enough relief, your physician might be able to recommend another medication or a remedy for the dryness.

COUPEROSE COMPLEXION

Couperose skin is highly sensitive facial skin characterized by dilated or expanded capillaries. A diffused redness, or erythema, is concentrated on the nose and cheeks. The capillaries can appear as tiny red dots or individual broken capillaries, or they can take on a spiderweb-like appearance, commonly called spider veins, a spider nevus, or spider telangiectasia. The tiny capillaries are quite visible through the skin's surface.

Causes of Couperose Skin

The classic appearance of couperose skin is, according to *Tabor's Cyclopedic Medical Dictionary,* "caused by capillary congestion, usually due to dilation of the superficial capillaries as a result of some nervous mechanism within the body, inflammation, or some external influence such as heat, sunburn, or cold." All skin types can suffer from a couperose condition, but those with fair skin and hair or sensitive, delicate, thin, or mature skin are most commonly affected. Smoking, excessive alcohol consumption, high blood pressure, temperature extremes, years of unprotected sun exposure, sunburn, and overzealous cleansing all contribute to couperose skin. Over the years vascular walls become damaged and can no longer handle the pressure of the blood flowing through them, so they break and leave you with a blotchy, ruddy complexion.

Prevention

Proper skin care is key to preventing the development or worsening of couperose skin. Wear sunscreen daily and avoid temperature extremes, or at least apply proper moisturizers prior to going outside. Avoid the causes of couperose skin listed above and pay attention to your health and stress level. It is amazing what nutritional neglect and environmental, work, and family stressors can do to your skin.

Furthermore, avoid alcohol-based toners, gritty facial scrubs, herbal steams, drying clay masks, and strong alpha-hydroxy and glycolic acid treatments, as these can be irritating if you suffer from this condition, even if it is just in its beginning stages.

Treatments

Couperose skin is a difficult condition to treat once it has developed, but with proper care you can help protect your skin against further deterioration and minimize the fragility of the capillaries.

Use gentle, mild products. You must use very gentle, fragrance- and color-free products to cleanse, tone, and moisturize. Lavender, rose, or German chamomile aromatic hydrosols make terrific anti-inflammatory and hydrating toners and aftershaves. They soothe the skin and reduce any feeling of surface dryness.

Exfoliate gently. Mix together equal parts of plain yogurt and finely ground sesame seed meal — 1 tablespoon (15 ml) is usually enough for one treatment. Gently massage the mixture onto your face, then rinse with cool water. This mild moisturizing and exfoliating mask is extremely gentle on the skin. It can be used once a week to clean fragile, sensitive skin and couperose complexions.

Supplement your diet. Increase your consumption of fresh, raw fruits and vegetables, especially those high in bioflavonoids (a class of phytochemicals found in the white inner rind of citrus fruits and in green and yellow vegetables, garlic, and onions). Bioflavonoids aid in strengthening capillary walls. Natural vitamin C with bioflavonoids might be a supplement to consider as well.

Consulting the Experts

See an Esthetician If: If you are in need of gentle, therapeutic cleansers and products to properly care for your couperose skin, your esthetician is the person to see. If you have couperose skin combined with another skin problem, she'll be able to guide you to the right product line.

See a Dermatologist If: If you'd like to eradicate those unsightly, red squiggly lines from your face, your dermatologist might recommend laser treatments to remove and destroy the defective surface capillaries.

CUTS, SCRAPES, AND OTHER IRRITATIONS

Let's face it — life can be hazardous! Everyday life is full of things that can bump, burn, scrape, grab, bruise, cut, bite, scratch, and poke your delicate skin. Minor injuries do and will happen, no matter where you are, leaving you with cuts, scrapes, and all sort of skin irritations.

Treatments for Irritations

Try the following easy-to-make, natural remedies that will soothe irritations and help prevent infection.

Note: If you've stepped on a nail or received a puncture wound from any metallic element, be sure to get a tetanus shot right away.

INFECTION CORRECTION SKIN CLEANSER

After cleansing the wound with this infection fighter, follow with Calendula Ointment (below) to help heal and relieve irritation.

1 cup (250 ml) hydrogen peroxide

20 drops tea tree essential oil

20 drops spike lavender essential oil

5 drops thyme (chemotype linalol) essential oil

Yield: 1 cup (250 ml)

To make: Combine all ingredients in an 8-ounce (250-ml) spray bottle or regular bottle, preferably glass. May store in a cool, dry cabinet for up to 1 year.

To use: Pour cool water over the affected area to clear it of debris, if necessary. Dab irritation with a cleanser-soaked cotton ball or gently pour the liquid directly onto the scrape, scratch, or insect bite. Use as needed to prevent infection, up to 3 times per day.

CALENDULA OINTMENT

This ointment helps heal and relieve a variety of skin irritations. In addition to soothing the usual assortment of cuts and abrasions, it makes an excellent preventive for diaper rash. Just apply to the little bottom after every diaper change to maintain fresh, healthy, soft skin. This ointment is also fabulous for dry, cracked hands and feet. Smells terrific, too!

1/2 cup (125 ml) all-vegetable shortening

10 drops calendula essential oil

10 drops everlasting or spike lavender essential oil

5 drops orange or lemon essential oil

Yield: 1/2 cup (125 ml)

To make: In a small bowl, allow the shortening to warm to room temperature. Add the essential oils. With a small whisk, whip ingredients together until thoroughly combined. Store in a glass or plastic container with a tight lid. Will keep, if refrigerated, for up to 1 year or up to 6 months if kept at room temperature.

To use: Clean the affected area and then apply the ointment. Use as necessary to help heal and prevent infection.

Consulting the Experts

See an Esthetician If: Everyday cuts and scrapes don't usually require the attention of a skin care specialist. However, if your esthetician carries a line of herb-based acne products, ask her if she sells a strong herbal astringent that contains either hydrogen peroxide or isopropyl alcohol. These particular products make good disinfectant washes and are handy to keep in first-aid kits.

See a Dermatologist If: If you notice that the affected area is not healing properly, or that it is red, sore, or filled with pus, you may have an infection. See your doctor as soon as possible to keep the infection from getting any worse.

DERMATITIS

Dermatitis comes from the Latin *dermatos,* meaning "skin," and *itis,* meaning "inflammation." According to *Taber's Cyclopedic Medical Dictionary,* dermatitis is an "inflammation of the skin evidenced by itching, redness, and various skin lesions." These various skin lesions can include blisters, pimples, lumps, dry skin, and scales.

Causes of Dermatitis

Dermatitis generally falls under one of two categories: irritant or allergic. *Irritant contact dermatitis,* the most common, can result in stinging, itching, redness, or burning sensations. It is an inflammation of the skin caused by contact with irritants to which you may be sensitive, such as abrasive cleansers, hair dyes, eye shadow, mascara, bar soaps, deodorants, moisturizers, wool fabrics, nickel (in jewelry), plant sap, and latex gloves. Construction workers frequently complain of rough, red, sore hands because they handle a variety of irritants — cement mix, fiberglass, acids, wood and metal chemicals, and paint, to name a few — and are at risk for developing occupational contact dermatitis. Healthcare workers, who frequently wash their hands, are at risk from constant exposure to water and detergents.

SKINFORMATION

Fragrance additives, whether natural or synthetic, cause more allergic contact dermatitis than any other ingredient. Preservatives are the second most common cause.

Allergic contact dermatitis is an inflammation of the skin that can result in swelling, redness, itching, hives, and oozing blisters, and is caused by a specific ingredient in a product to which you are allergic, such as lanolin, artificial colors, preservatives, fragrances, medicated creams, rubber, and glues. Upon your first contact with the potential allergen, a reaction is rare. However, repeated exposure will cause a reaction to occur even if the level of contact with the allergen is very low. This type of dermatitis has a tendency to spread to other parts of the body, away from the original contact site.

Prevention

If you are prone to allergies, and unsure of your reaction to a skin care product, try to find a tester bottle and place a little on your wrist or inner upper arm and leave it there for 8 to 12 hours. If all is still well, then you can generally feel safe about that product. Many times, though, it is not possible to test a product or item first, so proceed with caution. Take heart — most people can use common, everyday items without a problem, but if you're a sensitive type, take time to read labels and educate yourself about ingredients. Buy color-free, fragrance-free, and chemical-free products when available.

Treatments for Dermatitis

The symptoms of dermatitis can be quite irritating and annoying, so for temporary relief while your skin is healing, try the Comfrey Comfort Spray (see page 274), a cooling, soothing, herbal anti-inflammatory formula.

Consulting the Experts

See an Esthetician If: If you are reacting to a cosmetic product recommended by your esthetician, let her know. Sometimes she can return it to the manufacturer and refund your money. She'll also want to note your reaction in her records and may ask that you come in so that she can examine the irritated area and apply a soothing, anti-inflammatory treatment free of charge to ease your discomfort.

See a Dermatologist If: Dermatitis will usually clear up on its own once the irritant is removed, but if your dermatitis is not responding to home treatment, your doctor may wish to prescribe a cortisone or hydrocortisone lotion for short-term use. Antibiotics may be necessary if infection has set in.

COMFREY COMFORT SPRAY

Comfrey acts as an emollient, softening and comforting your skin. The peppermint and eucalyptus essential oils add a refreshing, cooling quality to the spray.

1 cup (250 ml) distilled water

1 teaspoon (5 ml) dried, chopped comfrey root, or 1 tablespoon (15 ml) fresh, chopped root

1/2 cup (125 ml) aloe vera juice

10 drops calendula essential oil

10 drops German chamomile essential oil

2 drops peppermint essential oil (optional)

2 drops eucalyptus essential oil (optional)

Yield: 1 1/2 cups (375 ml)

To make:
1. In a small saucepan, bring the water to a boil.
2. Add the comfrey root, then reduce heat and simmer, covered, to allow herb to decoct for 30 minutes.
3. Strain into a small bowl. Add aloe vera juice and essential oils. Stir thoroughly.
4. Pour liquid into a 12-ounce (375-ml) spray bottle or divide into two smaller bottles. If refrigerated, the spray will keep for approximately 2 weeks. If refrigeration is not possible, store in cool location and discard after 1 week.
To use: Shake well before each use and spray as often as necessary onto inflamed, itchy, burning, irritated areas.

DRY, FLAKY SKIN

Does your skin have small pores and a fine, thin texture? Does it soak up moisturizer like a sponge and keep begging for more? Does it get tight right after cleansing? Does it tend to become scaly, itchy, flaky, hot, red, sensitive to the touch, or parched? Well, my friend, you have dry skin, and this skin type ages faster than any other. Just what you wanted to hear, right?

Causes of Dry Skin

There are basically three types of dry skin: oil dry, water dry or dehydrated, and mature or aging skin. Oil-dry skin is caused by sebaceous glands that aren't functioning properly. Either they're lazy and sluggish or are simply failing to produce ample sebum. This type of dryness is usually inherited. Water-dry or dehydrated skin may be producing a sufficient amount of sebum but it's still dry on the surface due to a lack of moisture or water or as a side effect of medication. The third type of dry skin is caused by the natural aging process — a natural slow-down in the skin's regenerative capabilities. It just doesn't produce skin-softening sebum in the quantities that it did when it was younger.

Prevention

While you may not be able to prevent dry skin from occurring entirely, you can help keep it at bay by following these tips:

Avoid caffeine, smoking, and alcohol. They act as diuretics and are guaranteed to suck you dry.

Increase your water level. Drink up! Make sure to drink at least eight glasses of pure water a day to keep your skin and body properly hydrated. Drink more if you're super active.

Add oil to your bath. Add a tablespoon (15 ml) or so of almond, jojoba, olive, or hazelnut oil to your bath water after you've soaked for about 5 minutes. By soaking first, your skin gets plumped up by the water, then by adding the oil, it will seal in the absorbed moisture.

Protect your skin from the elements. Wind, sun, heat, cold, and dry office and airplane air can quickly cause or exacerbate the condition of dry skin. Apply a moisturizer before exposing your skin to these moisture-sapping villains. A lavender, rose, or German chamomile aromatic hydrosol sprayed onto your face, neck, hair, chest, and hands helps to keep your skin wonderfully refreshed and hydrated.

Limit hot water contact. Avoid long, hot showers and baths, especially during cold weather, as they dehydrate the skin. Warm showers and baths of short duration, though, are beneficial to dry skin. Also, limit bathing or washing your face to once a day, usually right before you retire. When you arise, apply a bit of herbal facial splash or toner or spritz your face (and body, if it needs treatment as well) with an aromatic hydrosol and you're ready to go.

Increase essential fatty acids (EFAs) in your diet. Chow down on salmon, herring, mackerel, bluefish, and sardines. These cold-water fish are a rich source of omega-3 fatty acids, which can help replace moisture in dry hair and skin. Also consider adding evening primrose oil to your diet. I take one 1,300 mg capsule daily — or every other day, depending on my body's needs — and my skin just blooms! Flaxseed oil supplementation is also beneficial — 1 tablespoon (15 ml) is the standard recommended dosage.

Buy humidifiers. They work wonders in restoring healthful humidity to your dry home or office environment.

Use only gentle cleansers. Avoid cleansers such as deodorant soaps and harsh abrasives. These can cause your skin to feel like a dried-out Thanksgiving turkey. Use a moisturizing soap, soap-free products, or a gentle grain-based cleanser.

Treatments for Dry Skin

Most dermatologists recommend plain old petroleum jelly as an effective barrier against moisture loss. It's messy, but it works. If you're adverse to applying petroleum products to your skin, try a nonpetroleum jelly product available in health food stores.

Give Dry Skin the One-Two Knockout

Perform these two treatments as often as 3 times per week.

Step 1: Exfoliate

This should always be the first step toward healing dry skin. Dead surface skin cells can, over time, build up and become unresponsive to lotions and creams. In order for your moisturizer to do its job, you must first get rid of this dead barrier. I like to use a gentle, grain-based scrub for my face. Mix 1 teaspoon (5 ml) ground oatmeal, 1 teaspoon (5 ml) white cosmetic clay, and 1 teaspoon (5 ml) ground flaxseed in a small bowl and add a bit of whole milk or cream. Stir everything together until a smooth paste forms and apply this to your face, gently massaging in a circular motion for about 1 minute. Rinse, and pat dry.

For my body I make a scrub that's a bit more abrasive. Combine 1–2 tablespoons (15–30 ml) salt with 1–2 tablespoons (15–30 ml) olive or quality vegetable oil in a small bowl. While in the shower, thoroughly scrub your entire body, making sure to spend a little extra time on the soles of the feet. Rinse and pat dry.

Step 2: Moisturize

After you've exfoliated, you're ready for moisture. Apply your favorite moisturizer to your face and body, or try good old vegetable shortening. (Shortening is typically made from 100 percent soybean oil and it soaks in rapidly — if you don't apply too much, that is!) I usually put my flannel gown and socks on after this and go to bed. You'll awaken with gloriously soft, smooth skin.

Consulting the Experts

See an Esthetician If: Your esthetician can tell you if your skin is oil dry or dehydrated and recommend treatment plans to bring it into balance. She is also a good source for gentle exfoliating creams and scrubs if you'd rather purchase them than make your own.

See a Dermatologist If: Generally a dry skin condition is relatively easy to remedy, but if you've tried everything to alleviate your dry skin and it's still not responding, perhaps you have something more serious and a visit to your doctor might prove prudent.

ECZEMA

Atopic dermatitis or atopic eczema, commonly referred to as simply eczema, usually begins in childhood and is hereditary. It mainly affects young children, teens, and young adults and is typically seen in families with a history of hay fever, asthma, or other allergies.

One of the early signs of infantile eczema is a localized, raised rash and swelling. As the disease progresses, redness and small blisters or vesicles form that can, over time, begin to ooze and crust. After age two, many children improve dramatically and have very few symptoms. That's good news, as infantile eczema can be hard on both the child and the parents — all the child wants to do is scratch, and so becomes irritable and unable to sleep; all the parents want to do is help their child and get some needed rest!

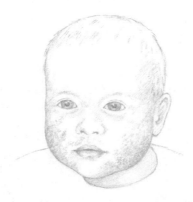

In infants, eczema is usually characterized by a localized, raised red rash on the face, elbows, or knees.

Eczema is not limited to childhood, though. It may go away temporarily and then flare up later in life. It may fluctuate seasonally as well. Eczema in adults tends to be dry, red to brownish gray, thickened, scaly skin. Intense itching causes some people to scratch until they bleed, which leads to infection, oozing, and crusting.

In infants, the skin rash usually begins on the face, elbows, or knees and may spread to other areas. Later in life, it can affect the elbow and knee folds, hands, ankles, wrists, neck, and upper chest.

SKINFORMATION

According to the National Eczema Association for Science and Education, "Individuals with atopic dermatitis have a lifelong tendency to suffer from various health problems:

- Dry, easily irritated skin
- Occupational skin disease — particularly hand dermatitis, causing considerable work loss
- Skin infections, especially staph and herpes
- Eye problems — cataracts and eyelid dermatitis
- Psychological disruption of family and social relationships

Causes of Eczema

The cause is actually unknown, but rest assured, eczema is not contagious. There are, however, many stressors or trigger factors that can aggravate the condition. These include cold weather, dry winter house heat and raw winter wind, emotional and physical stress, wool clothing, chafing from clothing, detergents, solvents, perfumes, dyes, heat and sweating, athlete's foot, herpes, pet dander, pollen, and food allergens.

Prevention

Here are a few tips to help prevent eczema flare-ups:

Moisturize, moisturize, moisturize! Unlike moist, soft, and flexible skin, dry skin is brittle and prone to cracking and infection, so keep your skin intact and your effective barrier healthy. Never let your skin dry out! Infused calendula oil (page 304) makes a particularly effective and soothing body moisturizer — massage into commonly affected areas as often as necessary.

Relax. Recognize your stressors, whatever they may be — work, family life, school, finances, or others — and learn to effectively manage them. The common reaction to stress in people prone to atopic dermatitis is red flushing and itching.

Know your genes. If eczema tends to run in your family, be prepared. Eat healthy, drink healthful immune strengthening herb teas (see Skin Ailment Assailment recipe, page 300), and avoid anything that can be a detriment to your health — smoking, lack of exercise, stress, soda, coffee, junk food, alcohol, and aggravating people and situations.

Supplement your diet. You need adequate intake of essential fatty acids and vitamins E and A to help keep your skin moisturized from within and win the battle against external dryness. In addition, make sure you are getting a good daily dose of vitamins C and B; zinc; and quercetin, a flavonoid, which may help prevent the formation of skin rashes.

Drink lots of fluids. Once again, I must reiterate: Be sure to drink plenty of fluids, especially water and fresh fruit and vegetable juices to keep your body hydrated.

SKINFORMATION

According to the National Eczema Association for Science and Education, "Eczema is one of the most common chronic skin diseases. Up to 10 percent of the population is affected, and there is no cure."

Treatments for Eczema

If you are fortunate enough to live near the ocean, take advantage of the healing properties of salt water. The cool ocean water will help relieve itching, inflammation, and general irritation caused by many forms of dermatitis, including eczema.

Evening primrose oil. According to Erica Lewis, author of "Essential Fatty Acids" in the July 1998 issue of *Les Nouvelles Esthetiques,* "Those with eczema may have an essential fatty acid deficiency. It is important for eczema sufferers to boost their dietary intake of the essential fatty acids because EFAs plump up the cell membranes and help repair old membranes and construct new ones. Eczema, psoriasis, dandruff, hair loss, dryness, and brittle nails respond to EFAs added to the diet."

OCEAN POTION

Landlocked readers for whom the ocean is just a distant summer's memory can enjoy a sea salt bath at home. If your eczema is weeping, oozing, and crusting, this treatment will help to soothe and cleanse the affected area(s), drain any infected sites, and aid in healing.

1 cup (250 ml) sea salt
5 drops carrot seed essential oil
5 drops calendula essential oil
2 teaspoons (10 ml) almond oil
1 tablespoon (15 ml) vodka, rum, or gin

Yield: 1 treatment

To make:

1. As the water runs into the tub, pour in the sea salt to dissolve.

2. As the tub is filling, combine the oils and alcohol in a small bowl, stirring rapidly to blend. Set aside.

To use:

1. Soak in the tub for 5–10 minutes to allow your skin to absorb moisture, then add the oils and alcohol and swish them throughout the water with your hands. These ingredients will soften and condition your skin.

2. Soak for 10–15 minutes longer, then pat dry and apply your favorite cream or lotion to seal in vital moisture. Note: Don't soak for longer than 20 minutes and only use warm water, as hot water will actually dehydrate your skin.

Clinical research has shown that evening primrose oil helps many people with arthritis pain, skin disorders, asthma, allergies, heart disease, and eczema. This seed oil is high in gamma-linolenic acid (GLA), an essential fatty acid that is needed by the body to produce the anti-inflammatory prostaglandins believed to combat these diseases and in turn strengthen cell membrane layers. Dosage recommendations range from 500 mg up to 3 to 4 grams per day, depending on the severity of the condition. Consult with your physician to find the right dosage for your particular situation.

Moisturizing treatments. With eczema, you must keep moisture in. Apply a good moisturizer immediately after showering or bathing. I recommend mixing vegetable shortening or a nonpetroleum jelly with a drop or two of lavender, calendula, German chamomile, or carrot seed essential oil and massaging the mixture onto your entire body. You can also use it to spot treat as necessary. This application creates a barrier to hold moisture in your skin that will help prevent further drying and itching of your eczema.

SOOTHING LICORICE TEA

In cases of skin irritations, including eczema, licorice can act as an anti-inflammatory agent upon the skin.

2 tablespoons (60 ml) dried licorice root
6 cups (1,500 ml) water

Yield: 6 cups, or 1 bath treatment

To make: Place the licorice and water in a saucepan, cover, and bring to a boil. Reduce heat and gently simmer, still covered, for 40 minutes. Strain.

To use: To relieve itching and irritation, add to a tub full of warm (not hot) water and soak for 10–15 minutes. You can also dab the tea directly onto itchy, dry patches of skin several times daily.

Another moisturizing treatment for irritated skin is to add ½ to 1 cup (125–250 ml) of finely ground or colloidal oatmeal to tepid bath water and have a good soak. This old-fashioned bath remedy is good for all types of dermatitis. A few cups of Soothing Licorice Tea (see page 282) added to bath water will also help relieve itching.

Consulting the Experts

See an Esthetician If: Your esthetician should carry a quality line of skin-enriching creams that will help seal in vital moisture and keep itching at bay. She may recommend a mild exfoliating gel to aid in gently removing the dead skin buildup that makes eczema unsightly.

See a Dermatologist If: If your eczema is not responding to home treatment, you may need to seek a doctor's advice. Medications such as topical or oral cortisone and antihistamines to control the itching are frequently useful for symptomatic relief, preferably as short-term treatments, as these drugs have undesirable side effects.

Another avenue to investigate is homeopathic medicine. Diseases such as arthritis, eczema, and psoriasis often respond positively to this type of complementary treatment. I highly recommend reading *Healing with Homeopathy,* by Dr. Wayne Jonas and Dr. Jennifer Jacobs.

EYE TIREDNESS

Are you a sight for sore eyes, or are your sore eyes a sight? Stressed eyes can be dry, itchy, irritated, red, burning, tired, or watery, and occasionally are surrounded by puffiness and dark circles. Sometimes these windows to your soul need a little pick-me-up. The treatments that follow should put the sparkle back.

Causes of Tired Eyes

Want to know a guaranteed way to look older quickly? Neglect your health and stress yourself out! Your eyes reflect the real you — a partier, an outdoors person, a sun worshiper, or a workaholic — and are the first part of your complexion to show signs of aging. The skin directly beneath the eyes does not contain sebaceous glands to lubricate it and is so very thin that a little neglect will immediately be reflected in and around your pretty peepers.

Many factors contribute to visual stress and unsightly eyes. A poor diet rich in simple carbohydrates and salt such as snack chips, candy, and fast food has a tendency to cause fluid retention in the eye area, and does nothing to nourish the rest of your body. Stress, lack of sleep, fluorescent light, dim light, sun, injury, alcohol, smoking, dry air, swimming in chlorinated pools, watching television, cosmetic fragrances, allergies, medication, repeated friction (such as eye makeup removal or contact lens placement), and sickness can lead to irritation, eye strain, dark circles, fine lines, and crow's-feet.

Dark circles, in particular, trouble many men and women. They make you look sick, tired, and older than your years. "In order to correct the problem of dark circles and other blemishes," states Dr. Victor Beraja, a board-certified plastic surgeon and author of "Eliminating Dark Eye Circles" *(Les Nouvelles Esthetiques,* March 1998), "one must know that cells beneath the epidermis called melanocytes produce the pigment that forms dark circles . . . when stimulated by a wide range of things, including . . . the gentle pull on the lids to insert contact lenses. . . . When this is repeated on a daily basis, for a long period of time, it can cause hyperpigmentation. Allergies and dry eyes work in a similar way. Irritation caused by these conditions lead a person to rub their eyes which again can cause hyperpigmentation. If the skin is excessively dry or sensitive to sun, even short exposure to the sun will irritate and stimulate the production of pigment. Of course, not all dark circles are caused by hyperpigmentation. Some circles are caused by swelling, poor circulation, and fluid retention."

Dark circles can also be the result of venous circulation, which is partially visible through the extremely thin skin beneath the eyes. Neither bleaching nor herbal treatments will work if this is the cause. Your best bet is makeup!

Prevention

To prevent the unsightly appearance of red, irritated eyes and dark circles, try these tips:

Wear sunscreen. Always wear sunscreen, either by itself or under your makeup — every day! Sunscreen helps prevent melanin formation within the thin, delicate skin around your eyes. Melanin is the dark pigment that can show up as unsightly dark circles.

Treat them gently. Don't pull or rub your eyes. Take eye makeup off gently using vegetable oil or a product specifically made to dissolve this type of makeup. Avoid using petroleum jelly or heavy cream near your eyes, as these can block the tear ducts and lead to water retention and puffy eyes.

Moisturize. Apply a water-based lotion or gel around the eye area once every day after cleansing to moisturize the delicate skin.

Take a break. Are you stuck behind a glaring computer screen or do you sit behind a desk grading papers or crunching numbers, all the while squinting your eyes? Give your eyes a break. Hour after hour of looking in one direction at small print and computer-screen light leads to eye irritation, tiredness, headache, and lazy eyes. Periodically stand up, stretch, and, ideally looking out a window, focus on something far in the distance, preferably a beautiful green tree or mountains. Without turning your head, look side to side several times, then up and down. Now, don't your eyes feel better?

Tune out. Don't be a TV addict. The glare from the screen is not good for your eyes.

Sleep. Pep up with plenty of sound sleep — one of the best eye (and body) beautifiers there is!

Treatments for Tired Eyes

Hydrosol spritzer. I sit at my computer writing for hours at a time and frequently get sore, dry, irritated eyes. My favorite treatment is to keep a bottle of lavender hydrosol handy and spritz my face and eyes with it as often as necessary. The liquid is so pure and gentle that I can spray it directly into my opened eyes. I find it extremely soothing. German chamomile and rose hydrosol work equally well.

Milk. For swollen eyelids, dip cotton balls or cosmetic squares into icy cold whole milk. Lie down, and apply soaked cotton to swollen eyelids and leave on for 5 to 10 minutes. The high fat content of whole milk provides a moisturizing treatment for the delicate, thin skin around your eyes.

Herbal compresses. My herbalist friend, Jean Argus, owner of Jean's Greens (see Resources), makes a delightfully refreshing herbal tea mixture called "For Your Eyes Only," containing eyebright, bilberry, chickweed, calendula, lavender, and goldenseal leaf. It's available in tea bags, which can be moistened with cool water and applied to irritated eyes, or made into an infusion to use as an eyewash or simply enjoyed as a nourishing beverage for your body.

You can make your own herbal compress with calendula or lavender using the Soothing Eye Compress recipe.

SOOTHING EYE COMPRESS

2 cups (500 ml) water
4 teaspoons (20 ml) freshly picked calendula flower petals or lavender buds (or 2 teaspoons [10 ml] dried)
Cosmetic cotton squares or large cotton balls

Yield: 6–8 treatments

To make:

1. Bring the water to a boil. Remove from heat, add the flowers, and cover.

2. Steep for 15 minutes, then place in the refrigerator and allow to cool for 1 hour.

3. Strain. Keep refrigerated and use within 4 days.

To use:

1. Moisten four cotton squares or balls with the herbal tea, squeezing out any excess liquid.

2. Lie down and place the cotton over your eyes — two pieces for each. Leave on for 5–10 minutes.

HERBAL EYEWASH

In her book, *The Herbal Medicine Cabinet,* published by Celestial Arts Press (Berkeley, CA: 1998), Master Herbalist Debra St. Claire recommends this recipe for general eye care. "This eyewash is for tired, strained eyes. It cleanses the tear ducts and stimulates circulation, which contributes to the tea's fame as a vision restorative." The eyewash should be made fresh for each treatment as it does not store well in the refrigerator.

1 cup (250 ml) distilled water
1 tablespoon (15 ml) dried eyebright
Glass eyecup (available in pharmacies)

Yield: 1 treatment

To make:

1. In a small saucepan, bring the water to a boil, then remove from heat. Add the eyebright, cover, and steep for 10 minutes.

2. While the eyewash is steeping, sterilize a glass eyecup by submerging it in boiling water for 5 minutes.

3. Strain the tea through a paper towel or doubled cotton cloth into a glass measuring cup. Cool until the tea is lukewarm.

To use:

1. Fill the eyecup with the cooled solution, pouring from the measuring cup into the eyecup (as opposed to dipping the eyecup in the solution).

2. Bend your head forward, place the eyecup firmly on your eye, then tip your head back, letting the solution wash the eye as you blink several times. It is helpful to hold a folded paper towel against your cheek to catch any drips.

3. Discard the used solution and refill the eyecup. Repeat the application to the same eye 3 separate times. Then resterilize the eyecup (this will prevent contamination of the second eye) and repeat the procedure on the other eye.

Tea. To reduce puffiness around the eyes, brew some regular black or green tea. They contain tannin, a natural astringent that helps to reduce swelling and puffiness. Chill the tea bags. Lie down with your head slightly elevated above your body and apply tea bags to your eyes. Rest with tea bags over closed eyes for approximately 20 minutes.

Fluid intake. Swollen eyes and dark circles can sometimes be the result of toxin buildup in the body as well as dehydration. Be sure to drink plenty of water daily in order to flush toxins and excess sodium from your body. When the body is dehydrated, the kidneys try to retain water, which results in puffiness and general ill health. The more water you drink, the less you will retain — it's a fact!

Over-the-counter products. Over-the-counter products containing skin-lightening hydroquinone or natural kojic acid have been proven effective in lightening hyperpigmented circles (those that are not hereditary) beneath the eyes. Caution: Always read the label of an over-the-counter product and make sure it specifically says that the product can be used around the eyes, as these creams can be quite irritating to some skin types, especially around the delicate eye area.

SKINFORMATION

The eyes blink about ten thousand times per day.

Consulting the Experts

See an Esthetician If: Your esthetician should be able to offer a few soothing eye treatments and recommend daily hydrating gels and light creams to ease the appearance of fine lines and wrinkles. Ask her if she offers a gentle exfoliating treatment to help lighten dark pigmentation under the eyes. If all else fails, I'm sure she'll be glad to sell you a quality makeup concealer to cover up your troubles!

See a Dermatologist If: If home remedies or a visit to your esthetician don't help soothe and beautify your eyes, then a visit to your dermatologist or eyecare specialist may be in order. Swelling, vision disorders, soreness, headaches, the feeling of roughness in your eyes when you blink, or watery eyes may be signs of internal problems or allergies.

HERPES SIMPLEX TYPE I

Herpes manifests as burning, tingling, itching, red, uncomfortable, tender blisters that appear on the lips and face. Some blisters are the size of pinheads and others may develop into much larger sores. The blisters begin to heal and form yellowish hard crusts, usually within a few days. Eventually this crust falls off and leaves the skin unscarred.

Causes

There are two types of the herpes simplex virus: HSV Type I, which most of us are familiar with, causes what is often called a cold sore or fever blister. HSV Type II causes genital sores and can be quite painful. I will discuss HSV Type I only.

Contrary to what their common names imply, cold sores and fever blisters are not caused by colds or fevers. Rather, they're caused by one of a group of viruses that is responsible for a number of other maladies such as mononucleosis, shingles, and chicken pox. Over 50 percent of the American population carry some form of the herpes virus in their nerve cells, where it quietly rests until set off by stress or illness.

SKINFORMATION

According to the American Academy of Dermatology, between 200,000 and 500,000 persons "catch" genital herpes each year and the number of Type I infections is many times higher. Prevention of this disease, which is contagious before and during an outbreak, is important.

Prevention

Here are some tips to help prevent this pesky virus from catching a foothold in your system:

Avoid undue stress. Flare-ups frequently occur when life is full of stressors from work, family, relationships, excessive heat and sunlight, illness, gastrointestinal upset, or respiratory infection. Anything that compromises the immune system can trigger a herpes outbreak.

Avoid spreading the contagion. To avoid catching or spreading the disease, do not kiss an infected person or kiss anyone while you are infected. Also, avoid sharing cups, eating utensils, or cosmetics and sexual contact with anyone that you suspect is infected.

Dry them out. If you're already infected, prevent a painful secondary infection. Don't get the sores wet, don't touch and pick at them, and don't cover them with bandages. They need to dry out, not be kept moist.

Treatments for Herpes

Currently, there is nothing that can totally prevent future herpes outbreaks and cure the underlying cause of the disease. All treatments are for symptomatic relief. There are several over-the-counter HSV Type I treatments to choose from. These formulations will usually relieve the pain, cool the burning, and aid in healing. Most come in either a lip balm or gel form; the active ingredients are generally phenol, camphor, menthol, and eucalyptus.

Soothing teas. Cold, strong lemon balm or peppermint tea can be applied to blisters that are inflamed and/or burning to help ease the pain and reduce the heat.

Supplement your diet. From a nutritional standpoint, the essential amino acid lysine has been shown to inhibit the growth of the herpes virus. Five hundred milligrams daily of lysine (available in most health food stores) is the common dosage taken between flare-ups with higher amounts taken during an outbreak. Lysine therapy does not have any side effects, but it would be prudent to check with your health professional first before adding it in supplement form to your diet. Some of the best food sources of lysine include salmon, canned fish, beef, goat and cow's milk, cooked mung beans, cheese, beans, cottage cheese, brewer's yeast, and shellfish.

On the other hand, the nonessential amino acid arginine has been shown to stimulate the growth of the virus. Arginine foods to avoid if you are prone to herpes outbreaks are: peanut butter, gelatin, chocolate, various nuts and seeds, and some cereals. Purchase a good nutrition guide so that you can educate yourself as to what foods are best to consume.

Support your immune system. Foods high in vitamins A, B, and C, zinc, and flaxseed oil all support immune system function and are beneficial to those suffering from HSV Type I.

Consulting the Experts

See an Esthetician If: Your esthetician may carry a good-quality herbal medicated lip balm specifically for minor cold sores or may be able to recommend a product — give her a call!

See a Dermatologist If: If you suffer from recurrent or severe Herpes Type I or II breakouts, your doctor may want to prescribe oral antiviral medications to reduce the number of attacks. Try to find a nutritionally oriented dermatologist who is familiar with complementary herpes treatments so that you may avoid drug usage if possible.

HERPES HEALING DROPS

To speed healing and help dry up oozing blisters, these antiviral herbal essential oil drops should provide relief.

2 tablespoons (30 ml) almond, jojoba, avocado, hazelnut, or soybean oil

2 drops blue cypress essential oil

2 drops eucalyptus essential oil

2 drops oregano essential oil

2 drops peppermint essential oil

2 drops tea tree essential oil

Yield: Approximately 1 ounce (30 ml)

To make: To a 1-ounce (30-ml) glass bottle, add all ingredients and shake vigorously. Allow oils to blend for 24 hours prior to use. Store bottle in a cool, dry place for up to 1 year.

To use: Apply the mixture by the drop, up to 3 times per day, to affected areas and gently massage into skin. Avoid ingesting this blend — do not let it drip into your mouth.

HIVES

I have a close friend who has a classic Type A personality. She works at two high-stress jobs a total of 60 to 70 hours per week, is a perfectionist, drinks an average of 5 cups of coffee a day, and teaches karate for 2 hours, 3 nights a week.

One summer day in 1996, during a very stressful and emotional period at her primary job, she began to develop intense itching on her torso, then on her neck and chest. The following day she woke up covered in roundish, red, raised blotches. She had no idea what was going on. Upon showing her husband her skin condition, he calmly told her she had a case of hives, commonly known as urticaria. She visited a dermatologist who confirmed the diagnosis.

Since then, whenever my friend finds herself under a heavy stress load, the itching begins and within minutes the pink swellings or wheals, as they are called, develop and last about 30 minutes, then disappear just as suddenly.

Hives can vary in size from as small as a pea to as large as 10 inches (25 cm) in diameter, usually itch, burn, or sting as they form, and fade away without a trace.

Causes of Hives

Angioedema, or hives that form around the lips, eyes, or genitals, generally result in excessive swelling, but tend to disappear within 24 hours. Acute urticaria is a term used to describe hives that last less than 6 weeks. This is the most common type of hives and usually appear in response to a food or drug allergy or infection. Hives that are caused by a food or drug allergy can, in addition to manifesting on the skin, result in the release of large amounts of histamines. Histamines are natural chemicals located in the skin that, when activated by an injury, allergic reaction, or other stressor, can cause flushing of the skin, swelling, tightness in the chest, wheezing, and a feeling of faintness. Chronic urticaria refers to outbreaks lasting for more than 6 weeks. Their cause is more difficult to pinpoint.

Physical urticarias are hives that develop from pressure, insect bites, vibration, cold, heat, exercise, or sunlight. Solar urticaria is a rare disorder in which hives develop within minutes after exposure to the sun, but disappear within hours.

Prevention

Hives are a very common malady, affecting approximately 10 to 20 percent of the population with at least one bout in their lifetime. Prevention can be difficult because you never know if you will be allergic to a new food or drug or if a new stressful situation in your life will cause hives. The best preventive is to avoid foods and drugs that are known systemic irritants and to minimize stress in your life.

Treatments for Hives

Find the cause, then eliminate it. According to dermatologists, this is the best treatment for hives. Unfortunately, this is not always the easiest of tasks to accomplish.

Soothing treatments. Treatments such as ice or cold aloe vera gel compresses can be applied directly to hives to help relieve the itching, shrink the wheals, and block the further release of histamines into your skin. One cup (250 ml) of baking soda and a few drops of lavender essential oil added to bath water will make a skin-relieving soak.

Relaxation therapy. In whatever form you seek — exercise, meditation, reiki, massage, reflexology, painting — relaxation therapy will aid in stress reduction, which is key to managing stress-induced hives.

Elimination diet. An elimination diet, guided by a doctor, nutritionist, or naturopath, can determine a particular food allergy and prevent future outbreaks of food-induced hives.

Supplement your diet. Vitamin C acts as a natural antihistamine, so make sure your diet includes ample amounts. You may want to supplement with 1,000 mg daily during an episode to help reduce the swelling.

Consulting the Experts

See an Esthetician If: If you need to unload the day's stress-es, book a facial or body treatment with your esthetician. An hour in her chair or on her treatment table will do wonders for your nerves. Ask her to add a few drops of lavender or German chamomile essential oil to her massage cream or perhaps to a mask and breathe deeply of the relaxing aroma.

If you have hives at the time of your appointment, ask her if she can apply a cold compress with a few drops German chamomile essential oil to help reduce the inflammation and relieve the itching.

See a Dermatologist If: An acute skin reaction to a food or drug can be life-threatening. If breathing becomes impaired, seek out emergency room treatment immediately. If you are hav-ing difficulty locating the cause of your hives, your doctor or naturopath may want to question you about food or drug aller-gies. Additionally, there are a number of infections that can cause hives, and these need to be ruled out as well. For tempo-rary relief, antihistamines can ease minor swelling and itching, but severe, recurrent hives may require an injection of epineph-rine (adrenaline) or a topical cortisone cream. Remember, the best possible course of treatment is to find the root cause of the hives and eliminate it, not to have to depend on drug therapy.

HYPERPIGMENTATION

"Out, out damned spot!" If only that's all it took — three magic words and those pesky skin discolorations would disappear for-ever. I'm afraid it's not that simple. You know what I'm talking about here — those flat, roundish, noncarcinogenic brown or reddish brown spots that, the older you get, frequently develop on the hands, arms, face, shoulders, feet, and legs. They're mainly a cosmetic, not health, concern.

Causes

Epidermal hyperpigmentation is the result of excess pigmenta-tion, or melanin accumulation, in the epidermal or dermal layer, and it is a harmless condition. Age, sun exposure, pregnancy, birth control pills, injury, chicken pox, shingles, acne scars, and heredity all play a role in the formation of hyperpigmented areas.

Chloasma gravidarum, or pregnancy mask, as it is commonly called, appears as brownish pigmentation areas on the face and neck. This uneven skin tone, due to fluctuating hormones and heightened sun sensitivity, usually disappears after delivery as the hormones settle back down.

Age spots or liver spots, also called lentigines, are caused by accumulated sun damage and may begin to appear in your thirties, depending upon the extent of past sun exposure. These discolorations often do not respond to commercial fade creams, but can be removed by your dermatologist if they really bother you.

Freckles are usually hereditary, can appear anywhere on the body, often darken with sun exposure, but tend to fade if you stay out of the sun. As a child, my cheeks and nose used to be covered with freckles, but now they've completely disappeared.

The skin on your pressure points, such as the elbows, knees, knuckles, palms, and soles of your feet, also tend to darken because of friction and sunlight.

Prevention

To prevent age spots from occurring and freckles from multiplying and darkening, stay out of the sun! The more you worship the sun, the more lovely brown spots your skin will probably sport. If your knees and elbows tend to darken easily, avoid leaning on your elbows as much as possible and avoid floor exercises that call for you to be on your knees.

Treatments for Hyperpigmentation

When I hit my early thirties, I suddenly developed an on-again/off-again case of very mild adult acne that left small, brownish purple spots on my cheeks and jawline after the pimples had healed. Unlike my teenage pimples that healed without a trace, these spots remained visible for approximately 6 weeks before fading. I found this quite aggravating and resorted to wearing makeup to cover them, until I found an at-home treatment that works like a charm. I still use it to keep my skin smooth and skin tone even.

Twice a week I use an unripened green papaya enzyme mask that softens and exfoliates. It's gentle enough to be used around my eyes, too. Two to three times a week, before I go to bed, I apply a mild glycolic acid gel to my just-cleansed skin, then follow with a light moisturizer if I need one. Both the mask and the gel are completely natural and can be purchased from most natural products suppliers (see Resources). You can use this combination of products wherever your skin needs to be lightened and the texture refined. I always wear a sunscreen to prevent damaging and darkening of my newly exfoliated skin.

Consulting the Experts

See an Esthetician If: For a bit more aggressive approach to lightening your skin, your esthetician has access to products such as alpha-hydroxy acid peels, enzyme peels, glycolic acids, and quality skin-lightening formulas that contain 1 or 2 percent hydroquinone (a depigmentation agent that suppresses melanin pigment formation within the upper layers of the skin). Many of her products have higher concentrations of natural acids and enzymes than those that are available to you over the counter and she is well educated in their proper use.

See a Dermatologist If: If your "spots" are a bit resistant to your home or esthetician's remedies, a dermatologist may prescribe topical agents such as retinoic acid (Retin-A) cream or alpha- and beta-hydroxy acids combined with prescription-strength hydroquinone. Dermatologists have had great success using these ingredients to even out patients' skin tone and give a smooth texture to the skin. Some people, though, are sensitive to hydroquinone and it should be used with caution.

If you have a brown spot or two that is changing color and/or size, please bring this to the attention of your doctor so that she can treat it accordingly.

PSORIASIS

Symptoms of this disease are raised, pinkish red, thick patches of skin, often covered with dry silvery gray scales, appearing on any part of the body, particularly the scalp, knees, elbows, fingernails, and lower back. As the top layer flakes off smaller red areas beneath are exposed, which then begin to grow, frequently becoming larger, thicker plaques or disc-shaped lesions. Psoriatic patches can itch, burn, or sting, depending on the severity of the disease. The disease generally develops slowly, typically followed by unexplained remissions and recurrences.

The symptoms can vary in severity from very mild, where the person doesn't realize he or she actually has the disease, to extremely debilitating psoriasis. As reported by the American Academy of Dermatology, "The most severe cases of psoriasis destroy the skin's protective functions, allowing the skin to lose fluids and nutrients; losing control of body temperature; making patients susceptible to infection; and possibly causing death." The National Psoriasis Foundation estimates that four hundred people die from psoriasis-related causes each year.

A small percentage of psoriasis suffers are afflicted with arthritis. Sometimes the arthritis symptoms improve as the patient's skin condition improves.

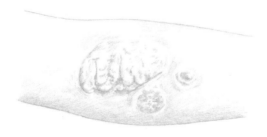

The elbow is one of the most common sites for the thick, scaly patches of skin that characterize psoriasis.

Causes of Psoriasis

Psoriasis gets its name from the Greek word for "itch." It is not contagious and tends to be hereditary. The disease is caused by abnormal skin cell production. Normal skin cells mature every 28 to 35 days, depending on age, and are sloughed off unnoticed. When skin is affected by psoriasis, skin cells mature in 3 to 4 days, causing them to pile up and resulting in thick skin plaques. Their red appearance is due to the rich blood supply feeding the rapidly multiplying new skin cells.

There are several biochemical reactions that prompt this abnormal skin cell growth. They can be triggered by injury to the skin, some types of infection, a drug reaction, physical or emotional stress, or a surgical incision. Many herbalists suggest that it's a toxic liver or anxiety that causes psoriasis.

Prevention

If your parents suffered from psoriasis, chances are likely that you will too. But you can take measures to help prevent the disease from progressing. Eat a diet that is high in vitamins A, B, C, D, and E, zinc, and onions and garlic for their sulfur content. Supplements such as evening primrose oil or borage oil and supplement forms of the vitamins and minerals mentioned may be a prudent measure.

My skin care mentor, licensed esthetician Lozetta DeAngelo, believes that psoriasis is a stress-induced disease and suggests using stress reduction methods such as hypnosis, exercise, deep breathing, and yoga. She also says that due to today's agribusiness practices, our foods are not what they used to be nutritionally, thus our bodies suffer from a lack of vital nutrients and our skin reflects this deficiency.

Treatments for Psoriasis

Sunshine. The sun greatly aids in the healing of psoriasis lesions, but exposure to the sun can lead to premature aging, age spots, leathery skin, and possibly skin cancer. A few minutes spent in the sun in the morning and evening may prove beneficial, with minimal side effects, or you can apply sunscreen to all areas of your body except those affected by psoriasis and stay outside a bit longer.

Consulting the Experts

See an Esthetician If: The assistance your esthetician can provide is palliative at best. She is your best source, other than your dermatologist, for efficient moisturizing creams to help keep your psoriasis patches soft and flexible, minimizing dryness, cracking, and bleeding.

See a Dermatologist If: If your psoriasis condition continues to worsen, despite self-help remedies and nutritional therapy, see your dermatologist. She or he can prescribe relatively safe topical treatments such as tar and cortisone creams for a mild to moderate case, or oral medications for a more severe case. Be aware that these drugs are not without serious side effects. In my opinion, as with any disease condition, it is always best to seek alternative therapies before resorting to potentially harmful drug treatment.

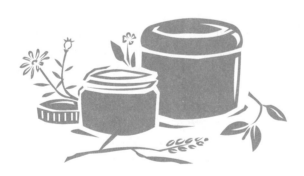

SKIN AILMENT ASSAILMENT TEA

All herbs in this formula are in dried form. It can be prepared as either a tea or a tincture.

4 parts burdock root
2 parts sassafras root bark
2 parts dandelion root
1 part Oregon grape root
1 part cinnamon bark granules (optional in tincture recipe)
1 part calendula flowers
1 part oat flowering tops
1 part echinacea herb or root
1 part nettle leaf
1 part cleavers herb

Tea yield: ½ gallon (2 liters)
Tincture yield: Approximately 2–3 cups (500–750 ml), depending on how finely chopped the herbs are

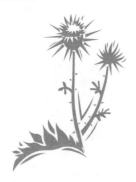

To make:
Mix all herbs in a large bowl. Store in a tin, plastic tub, or zip-seal plastic bag in a dark, dry cabinet or drawer. Will keep for up to 1 year.

To prepare a tea:
1. Put 8 tablespoons (120 ml) of the herb mixture in a pot with ½ gallon (2 liters) of water.

2. Bring to a low simmer (do not let it boil!) and cook, covered, for ½ hour. Turn off heat and let stand for at least 2 hours — all day would be fine.

3. Pour the mixture into a widemouthed jar and refrigerate. Each batch will last for 3–4 days.

To use the tea:
Strain off each cup as needed. If your condition is severe, you could try 3–4 cups of tea per day. If you experience discomfort as the body begins to release toxins, reduce the amount (or stop altogether) until you are reasonably comfortable again, then begin to slowly increase your daily intake. Do not expect dramatic results until you have been on this protocol for at least 3–4 weeks (some individuals may notice changes more readily).

To prepare a tincture:

1. Place 3 cups (750 ml) of the herb mixture in a wide-mouthed quart (liter) jar. Cover with vodka (100 proof is best), with a mixture of 50 percent pure grain alcohol and 50 percent distilled water, or with organic vinegar. The liquid should be about 1 inch (2.5 cm) above the level of the herbs.
2. Cover tightly. Shake several times a day for at least 2 weeks, preferably 3–4 weeks.
3. Finally, strain through a cheesecloth or press with a potato ricer. Strain again into a dark glass bottle.
4. From this master bottle, you may decant into a 2- or 4-ounce (60- or 125-ml) dropper-top bottle for easy dosing. Be sure to label all bottles and keep them out of reach of children.

To use the tincture:

Half a teaspoon, 3 times a day in water or juice may be a good starting dose for a 150-pound (68-kg) adult. Adjust the amount for your constitution and size. Decrease amount as you begin to see results.

HOW MUCH IS A "PART"?

A part can refer to any amount. It can mean teaspoons, tablespoons, cups, quarts, gallons, and so on. You assign a meaning to it depending upon how much formula you want to make. Half of a part will be half of whatever increment you are using. For instance, if in this recipe you decided that part would mean "cups," you'd have a whole lot of skin tea formula. If you decided that it would mean "teaspoons," then you'd be making enough for approximately 15 cups of skin tea, as the recipe calls for a total of 15 parts of herbs and it usually requires 1 teaspoon of dried herb per cup of boiling water. Understand?

COMFREY/CALENDULA HEALING SALVE

Formulated for treatment of psoriasis, this salve is also useful as a cuticle conditioner and can be used to soften dry feet, knees, elbows, and hands. This salve can also be used to heal and fade the appearance of scars.

- 1 quart (1 l) extra-virgin olive oil
- 3/4 cup (180 ml) dried comfrey leaves
- 3/4 cup (180 ml) dried calendula flowers
- 3/4 cup (180 ml) freshly wilted St.-John's-wort flowers
- 1/2 scant cup (125 ml) dried plantain leaves
- 1 teaspoon (5 ml) myrrh gum resin powder
- 1 tablespoon (15 ml) vitamin E oil
- 1/2 cup (125 ml) beeswax

Yield: Approximately 1 quart (1 liter)

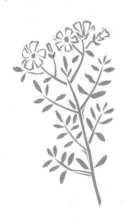

To find the flowers:

The St.-John's-wort flowers are most potent when fresh, so the flowers used in this recipe must be freshly picked. If you don't grow St.-John's-wort in your garden, you'll have to wildcraft some blossoms for this recipe. St.-John's-wort can be found blooming in poor soil just about everywhere. It grows in masses up to 3 feet (1 m) tall and has a cheery, bright, small yellow flowers. Check a local flower guide to help you properly identify the plant. To help keep wild-growing populations of St.-John's-wort thriving, harvest just what you need, and don't harvest the entirety of any one population — leave enough that the plants will be able to regenerate. Do not harvest flowers from areas where pesticides are used or from the pollutant-filled areas near highways.

To make:

1. Add the olive oil to a slow cooker or 3-quart (3-l) saucepan and warm over the lowest possible heat setting. You want the oil to become just nicely warm — do not let it simmer! Add all of the ingredients except the vitamin E and beeswax. Stir thoroughly to coat the herbs with the oil and leave the heat for 12–24 hours, uncovered, stirring occasionally.

2. Strain the herbs through a potato ricer or mesh strainer lined with panty hose into a fresh bowl. Press the herbs in the strainer to squeeze out all of the oil. If you notice lots of particulate matter in the bottom of the bowl, you may want to restrain the liquid, but it's not necessary. Discard the spent herbs in your compost or garden.

3. In a 2-quart (2-l) saucepan, melt the beeswax over very low heat, then add the herbal oil. Stir to blend thoroughly, then remove from heat. You should have a slightly warm, golden-greenish oily liquid.

4. Stir in the vitamin E, which acts as a preservative. This recipe makes a large amount of salve, so you may want to pour it into four 8-ounce (225-g) jars or eight 4-ounce (115-g) jars for easier storage. If refrigerated, the salve will last for approximately 1 year; if left at room temperature, it should be used within 6 months.

To use:

Apply this salve as often as necessary to soothe, soften, and heal dry, crusty psoriatic patches.

WILTING FLOWERS

Some herbal treatments, such as the Comfrey/Calendula Healing Salve (on page 302) and Calendula Oil (on page 304), call for "freshly wilted" flowers. Fresh and wilt may seem a contradiction of terms, but there is a reason for it: A day of wilting allows a large proportion of the water that flowers contain to evaporate, maximizing the potency of the preparation they'll be used in.

To wilt freshly picked flowers, spread them onto an herb-drying screen or lay them on newspaper that is covered with a layer of paper towels. Keep the flowers in a place that gets plenty of air circulation but is out of the sun and away from dirt. After 24 hours, the flowers should be nicely wilted and a large proportion of the water they contain should have evaporated.

CALENDULA OIL

This calendula-infused oil makes a soothing, gentle treatment for the itchy, sometimes painful symptoms of psoriasis, eczema, and even everyday rashes. It also makes a wonderful bath and massage oil.

2 cups (500 ml) dried calendula flowers (or 3 cups [750 ml] fresh-ly wilted flowers — see page 303)
1 quart (1,000 ml) extra-virgin olive oil
1 tablespoon (15 ml) vitamin E oil

Yield: Approximately 1 quart (1 liter)

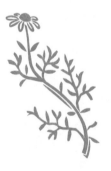

To make:

1. Pour the olive oil into a slow cooker or large saucepan and warm over the lowest possible heat setting. You want the oil to be just nicely warm, or about 125˚F (50˚C) — don't let it simmer. Add the flowers and stir to coat all the petals. Leave over heat for 12–24 hours, uncovered, stirring every few hours.

2. Strain the mixture through a mesh strainer lined with panty hose, catching the herbal oil in a bowl placed below. Press the remaining oil out of the flowers. (You can compost the spent flowers in your garden.)

3. Mix the vitamin E oil into the herbal oil. Store the oil in the refrigerator and use within 6 months.

To use:

Rub right into any itchy, painful, dry spots; add a couple of tablespoons (30 ml) to a warm bath; use as a massage oil for normal-to-dry skin; or add to massage and facial oils as a soothing, moisturizing agent.

APPENDIX:
A Guide to Ingredients

⌄⌄⌄⌄⌄

This chapter is a descriptive journey through my "green world." I use all of the natural ingredients that follow in the personal care products I make for myself and my friends, family, and clients. By adopting at least a few of these ingredients into your skin care repertoire, you will be educating yourself about what you put in and on your body. Only you can take control of your skin's health!

BASE OILS

Base oils are derived from nuts, seeds, vegetables, and fruits. They have mild therapeutic properties, but as the name implies, they are most often used as a base or carrier oil to which essential oils and herbs are added when making oils, lotions, or creams.

The best oils to purchase for skin care purposes are cold- or expeller-pressed, as they are not extracted at extremely high temperatures and/or with a chemical solvent. (Exposure to high temperatures and chemical solvents can destroy natural flavors, aromas, antioxidant properties, and beneficial trace minerals and vitamins.) Cold-pressed oils are processed at a relatively low temperature (150–250˚F, or 65–120˚C). Expeller-pressed oils have been mechanically pressed from the nut, seed, fruit, or vegetable from which it is derived. Cold- and expeller-pressed oils, by the way, are also highly recommended for use in cooking and salad dressings, as they have a better flavor and higher nutritional value than conventionally processed oils.

Base oils, with the exception of avocado, hazelnut, jojoba, and extra-virgin olive, tend to become rancid if stored at room temperature for more than 4 to 6 months; they should be refrigerated. The oils described below should have only a trace of fragrance, if any at all. If the oil has a strong or "off" smell (with the exception of olive oil), then it's probably

⌄⌄⌄⌄⌄

PRESERVATION

To prolong the shelf life of your base oil, pierce eight to ten vitamin E capsules. Add the contents of the capsules to every 8 ounces of oil.

▲▲▲▲▲

old. Purchase base oils through reputable mail-order suppliers (see Resources) or better health food stores with a high inventory turnover. Don't hesitate to return the product if it is bad.

ALMOND OIL

Description: A clear to very pale yellow oil pressed from sweet almond seeds (kernels). Full of vitamins and minerals. Reasonably priced and widely available.

Uses: From massage oils to lotions, creams to masks, almond oil is good for all skin types, especially dry, inflamed, or itchy skin. A first-rate, all-purpose oil.

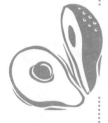

AVOCADO OIL

Description: A clear, medium to dark green oil derived from the fatty fruit pulp. Rich in protein, vitamins, and fatty acids. A very stable oil with a long shelf life. Moderately priced and sometimes difficult to find.

Uses: Especially good blended with other base oils and used as an after-bath body or facial oil — use 1 part avocado oil to 10 parts other base oils. The perfect, nourishing oil for dull, lifeless, dry, and devitalized skin; eczema; and psoriasis.

BORAGE SEED OIL

Description: A pale yellow oil pressed from the seeds. Very rich in beneficial GLA (gamma linolenic acid), vitamins, and minerals. Expensive, but worth it.

Uses: Taken internally, borage seed oil lessens PMS symptoms and helps to lubricate joints and skin. When blended with avocado, jojoba, hazelnut, or almond oil, it is used externally to treat eczema, psoriasis, and signs of premature aging. Dilute with other base oils using a 1 to 10 ratio.

CASTOR OIL

Description: A very thick, clear to slightly yellow oil processed from the seeds of an annual shrub. Extremely moisturizing. Inexpensive and easy to find.

Uses: I like it for the staying power and shine it provides to my lip balm and gloss recipes. Particularly good for softening rough, dry heels, knees, elbows, and patches of eczema and psoriasis.

COCONUT PALM OIL

Description: Expressed from coconut meat, this white semisolid fat melts at room temperature. Widely available and inexpensive.
Uses: Excellent as a massage or bath oil or when used in lotions and creams. A mild, gentle oil, good for sensitive and infant skin.

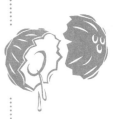

HAZELNUT OIL

Description: A clear, pale yellow oil derived from the pressed kernel, hazelnut oil has a mild, nutty fragrance. High in vitamin E and fatty acids. It has a light, penetrating quality that makes it good for all skin types. Usually only available through mail-order suppliers (see Resources), moderately priced.
Uses: One of the best base oils used in face creams and lotions because of its lightness and stability (it is not prone to rancidity). Especially good for aging skin.

JOJOBA OIL

Description: Actually a liquid plant wax, this clear, yellow oil is pressed from the seeds. The thick oil closely resembles human sebum in consistency. Will not become rancid; hardens in cold weather. Expensive, but relatively easy to find.
Uses: Good for inflamed skin, eczema, psoriasis, rough or dry skin, and acne. Penetrates easily and is very compatible with human skin.

OLIVE OIL

Description: A clear green oil with a strong olive fragrance taken from the first pressing of ripe olives. High in vitamin E. Moderately priced, widely available. Be sure to choose the extra-virgin variety.
Uses: Though a very high-quality cosmetic oil, I rarely use it, except when combining with salt to make body scrubs or salves, because of its overpowering fragrance and color.

ROSEHIP SEED OIL

Description: Clear, reddish in color, derived from the seeds of the ripened fruit of *Rosa rubiginosa* (commonly known as Rosa Mosqueta). Extremely high in essential fatty acids. Expensive and usually only available from better health food stores or mail-order suppliers (see Resources).

Uses: Used with much success in treatments for skin damage that has resulted in premature aging, dehydration, wrinkles, or scars. Highly recommended for mature, dry, and sun-damaged skin.

Contraindication: Should not be used on skin that is oily or acneic.

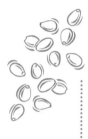

SESAME OIL

Description: Derived from the pressed seeds, this clear, golden oil is rich in vitamins A and E and protein. It's a very stable base oil, meaning that it has a long shelf life.

Uses: Used in sunscreens, salves, and lotions. Superb as a body oil for normal-to-dry skin.

Note: Do not use the toasted varieties of sesame oil in your skin care products.

SOYBEAN OIL

Description: A clear, yellow, highly refined, widely available, inexpensive oil. Commonly found in grocery stores under the label of "vegetable oil." Check the ingredients panel and it should read "100 percent soybean oil."

Uses: A terrific massage oil. Penetrates readily with no greasy residue. Not my number one choice, though, because of the chemical residues found in most brands as a result of processing, but can be used in a pinch. Try to find an organically produced soybean oil.

ESSENTIAL OILS

Essential oils are steam distilled from flowers, roots, barks, seeds, leaves, resins, or twigs, or are pressed from citrus rinds. Unlike a vegetable or nut oil, an essential oil is not actually an "oil" because it does not contain fatty acids and is not prone to rancidity. For extraction purposes, low pressure and low temperature methods ensure top-quality fragrance and therapeutic value. I purchase my essential oils from a handful of companies I've come to know and trust (see Resources). Their oils are of superior quality and suitable for aromatherapeutic skin care treatments. Many health food stores and herb shops also carry quality essential oils.

An essential oil is the life-force or the "soul" of the plant. Each precious, aromatic, highly volatile, concentrated drop of an essential oil contains plant hormones and organic chemical compounds that regenerate and oxygenate the skin. They are important to include in therapeutic skin care treatments because their small molecular structure allows them to easily penetrate into the dermis to nourish, rejuvenate, and regenerate skin cells. Unlike most ingredients in a moisturizing cream, which stay primarily on the skin's surface, essential oils are absorbed all the way down to the subcutaneous tissue layer.

BLUE CYPRESS (CALLITRIS INTRATROPICA)

Description: Distilled from the branches and leaves of an Australian tree — very rare, but exceptional! The oil is clear, medium blue-green in color, and smells like musty, wet, forest-floor leaves, but when applied to warm skin develops a mellow, sandalwood-like fragrance. Quite wonderful, really!

Cosmetic Properties and Uses: Superior essential oil for dry or mature skin. Contains antiviral properties. Can be used as an effective replacement for essential oil of sandalwood, which is rapidly becoming endangered. Excellent treatment for ridding your skin of warts.

CALENDULA (CALENDULA OFFICINALIS)

Description: Derived from the petals of the beautiful orange or yellow flower. The oil is clear, deep orange in color and has a heavy, intoxicating, herbal fragrance.

Cosmetic Properties and Uses: Antiseptic, antifungal, and anti-inflammatory. Good for healing scar tissue, burns, bruises, acne, insect bites, and cuts. Gentle enough for young children. I normally add a few drops to every cosmetic I make or purchase. One of my favorites!

CARROT SEED *(DAUCUS CAROTA)*
Description: Distilled from carrot seeds, this essential oil is clear, yellowish-orange in color, and smells slightly spicy-sweet, reminiscent of fresh carrots.
Cosmetic Properties and Uses: High in beta-carotene. A very nourishing, vitalizing, and restorative oil. Stimulates skin elasticity. Good for all skin types, especially wrinkled, normal-to-dry, and sagging skin.
Contraindication: Should not be used by epileptics or women who are pregnant.

CHAMOMILE, GERMAN *(MATRICARIA RECUTITA)*
Common Names: Blue chamomile, wild chamomile
Description: An intensely deep blue oil, distilled from the flowers of this lacy, delicate, pretty plant. The heavy chamomile fragrance tends to overpower any formula it is added to and the blue color also dominates, turning many cosmetics blue-green.
Cosmetic Properties and Uses: High in azulene content. Extremely soothing and healing to irritated, couperose, normal-to-dry, and sensitive skin. A strong anti-inflammatory and antifungal natural medicine. Powerful relaxant. Beneficial for acne when blended with spike lavender and everlasting essential oils.

EUCALYPTUS *(EUCALYPTUS DIVES)*
Common Name: Blue peppermint eucalyptus
Description: A clear, pale yellow-to-green oil with a refreshing menthol/balsam/camphor-like fragrance. It is distilled from the leaves of this plant.
Cosmetic Properties and Uses: Recommended in formulas for balancing the production of excess sebum in oily or acneic skin. Used as an inhalant to relieve chest congestion.
Contraindication: Should not be used by epileptics or women who are pregnant.

ESSENTIAL OIL STORAGE TIPS

- Because essential oils can be harmful if ingested, it is important to store them out of reach of children and pets.

- To prolong the shelf life of an essential oil, do not store the oil in a bottle with a rubber top. The strong vapors emitting from the oil will gradually weaken the rubber and allow air to enter the bottle, and the precious volatile healing properties will evaporate prematurely. If you intend to keep a particular bottle of oil longer than 60 months, seal it with a plastic screw-top cap and reserve the dropper for that essential oil only.

GERANIUM, ROSE *(PELARGONIUM X ASPERUM, GRAVEOLENS)*

Description: A clear, pale greenish-yellow oil distilled from the leaves of this beautiful plant. Has a strong, earthy, minty-sweet, uplifting, almost roselike aroma.

Cosmetic Properties and Uses: Good for normal and normal-to-oily skin. Has mild astringent properties. Helps to heal burns, abrasions, ulcers, and acne when combined with spike lavender and rosemary.

EVERLASTING or IMMORTELLE *(HELICHRYSUM ITALICUM)*

Description: A clear, yellowish oil distilled from the whole plant. Highly aromatic with a currylike smell.

Cosmetic Properties and Uses: Very strong anti-inflammatory, antibacterial, and antifungal. Said to be even more potent than German chamomile. Indicated for healing bruises, open wounds and cuts, varicose veins, acne, eczema, and psoriasis. Very soothing. Stimulates new cell formation.

INULA *(INULA GRAVEOLENS)*

Description: A clear-to-pale green oil distilled from the flowers with a medicinal, sweet, camphorlike aroma.

Cosmetic Properties and Uses: Ideal for oily, acneic, overly clogged skin. Loosens sebum. Highly antibacterial and mucolytic. Works well blended with eucalyptus and spike lavender.

Contraindication: Should not be used by epileptics or women who are pregnant.

JUNIPER BERRY *(JUNIPERUS COMMUNIS)*

Description: A clear, pale yellow oil distilled from the berries or small branches of this evergreen shrub. Has a sweet balsam, woody fragrance.

BUYER BEWARE

Essential oil production is a labor-intensive and material-expensive project. It takes approximately 500 pounds of rosemary to produce 1 pound of oil. Jasmine absolute, one of the most expensive essential oils (retails for three to six hundred dollars per ounce), requires approximately eight million hand-picked blossoms, harvested before sunrise, to produce just over 2 pounds of oil. A high-quality oil is expensive, but it is worth it. Unfortunately, there are some pretty low-quality oils out there, so you need to know the distinguishing features of a quality essential oil.

1. Look for "g & a" (genuine and authentic), "vintage," or "organic" on the label, or ask for therapeutic or pharmaceutical grade oils. These essential oils have been steam distilled at low temperatures. You will pay more for this type of processing, but you'll be ensured of a pure, effective product.

2. Essential oils are highly volatile and will evaporate quickly. Place a drop or two of essential oil on a sheet of plain paper, spread it around a bit, and leave it alone for 5 to 10 hours. A real essential oil will evaporate and will not leave a stain, or perhaps a very minor one. A vegetable oil will leave a greasy stain, as potato chips do if placed in a brown paper bag.

3. Vegetable oils have a greasy feel; essential oils do not. Rub a little vegetable oil between your fingers and notice how slippery it is. Now rub a drop of essential oil between the fingers of your other hand. It may initially feel greasy, but the essential oil will quickly be absorbed or feel more like water. If the essential oil feels like vegetable oil, it probably has been diluted.

Cosmetic Properties and Uses: A good antiseptic and cleansing addition to products for oily skin or eczema. Is frequently used in massage oil formulas for cellulite because of its strong diuretic action.

Contraindication: Avoid if you have a history of kidney problems, are pregnant, or are epileptic.

LAVENDER *(LAVANDULA ANGUSTIFOLIA)*

Description: A clear, yellow-green oil steam-distilled from the fragrant blossoms. Highly valued as a potent healing agent and floral perfume additive.

Cosmetic Properties and Uses: Good for all skin types. One of the few oils that can be used "neat," or undiluted. Powerful relaxant and a strong yet gentle antiseptic; effective as a remedy for sunburn, bee stings, muscle cramps, burns, and insomnia. Safe for everyone, including infants and pregnant women.

LEMONGRASS *(CYMBOPOGON CITRATUS)*

Description: A clear, yellowish brown liquid distilled from the grassy leaves of this plant. Has a pleasant lemony fragrance.

Cosmetic Properties and Uses: Used in cleansers and moisturizers for normal-to-oily skin because of its mild astringent property. Also good for sagging, devitalized smoker's skin — helps to eliminate wastes.

Contraindication: Do not use on sensitive or irritated skin.

ORANGE, SWEET *(CITRUS SINENSIS)*

Description: A clear, pale-to-vibrant orange oil with a strong, uplifting, orangelike fragrance. Extracted from the fruit rind.

Cosmetic Properties and Uses: Recommended for all skin types except very dry. Slightly astringent.

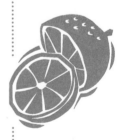

Contraindication: Can cause skin to become photosensitive (abnormally reactive to sunlight). Do not use if you are pregnant or epileptic.

OREGANO *(ORIGANUM COMPACTUM, O. VULGARE)*

Description: Distilled from the leaves and stems of these highly aromatic members of the mint family. It has an oregano/mint fragrance. Very warming on the skin with a clear, yellow to earthy brown color.

Cosmetic Properties and Uses: Powerful antiseptic and antiviral. Good for treating warts, insect bites, fungal infections, and general skin infections.

Contraindication: This essential oil is a skin irritant and must be well diluted. Avoid if you are pregnant or epileptic.

PEPPERMINT MITCHAM *(MENTHA X PIPERITA)*

Description: A clear-to-pale green oil distilled from the stems and leaves. This particular type of peppermint essential oil has a very sweet, almost candylike aroma, without the sharp bite that other peppermints have. If "Mitcham" is unavailable, regular peppermint is fine. Mitcham is my personal favorite.

Cosmetic Properties and Uses: Very refreshing, cooling, and astringent when made into a facial toner or body splash or cleanser for normal-to-oily skin. An excellent antiseptic when blended with tea tree and orange essential oils.

Contraindication: A potential skin irritant if used in large amounts. Do not use if you are pregnant or epileptic.

ROSEMARY (*ROSMARINUS OFFICINALIS,* CHEMOTYPE VERBENON)

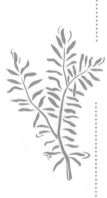

Description: This oil is a colorless, clear liquid. Has an earthy, strong fragrance with a dominant camphor/eucalyptus note. Distilled from the stems and leaves of this plant.

Cosmetic Properties and Uses: Known for stimulating new cell formation. Can benefit all skin types, and particularly good in regenerative, nurturing skin care formulations for wrinkled, devitalized, aging, acneic, burned, scarred, or sun-damaged skin.

Contraindication: Do not use if you are pregnant or suffer from epilepsy or high blood pressure.

SPIKE LAVENDER *(LAVANDULA SPICA)*

Description: A clear, pale yellowish green oil distilled from the flowers. Highly aromatic, floral, with a clean, lavender fragrance.

Cosmetic Properties and Uses: Helps to normalize and balance the skin. Good for all skin types. Also an effective antiseptic for burns, cuts, and insect bites. Makes a nice addition to a relaxing massage oil formula.

Contraindication: Avoid during pregnancy or if you suffer from epilepsy.

WHAT'S A CHEMOTYPE?

Plants of the same botanical species can produce essential oils of distinctly different compositions, or chemotypes. The reason for this is not completely understood, but factors such as where the plant is grown and its genetic lineage can contribute to this phenomenon, known as chemical polymorphism.

For example, as you can see under the listing for rosemary, the botanical Latin identification is followed by a chemotype identification, specifically verbenon. This is the chemical component, or chemotype, most characteristic for that species of plant. I've chosen the verbenon chemotype because it is a very gentle, nonirritating essential oil that is a staple for high-quality skin care preparations.

Only the labels of superior quality, pharmaceutical or aromatherapeutic grade essential oils will offer these chemotype distinctions. Try to locate these specific types of essential oils so that you can achieve maximum results with your homemade preparations.

— Adapted from *Aromatherapy Course*, Part I,
Essential Oils, 2nd edition, by Dr. Kurt Schnaubelt

TEA TREE *(MELALEUCA ALTERNIFOLIA)*
Description: A clear, pale yellow oil that is distilled from the leaves of an Australian tree. Has a pungent, balsam/camphor medicinal scent.
Cosmetic Properties and Uses: Powerful antibacterial, antifungal, and antiseptic. Helps heal acne, open wounds, cuts, ulcers, and infections. Makes a good addition to cleansers for acneic skin.

THYME (*THYMUS VULGARIS*, CHEMOTYPE LINALOL)
Description: A clear-to-yellowish oil with less "bite" than other, hotter thyme oils, this is a softer, nonirritating variety of thyme. Distilled from the branches, leaves, and flowers. Has a sweet/spicy, fresh scent.
Cosmetic Properties and Uses: A strong antiseptic. Highly recommended in treatments for infectious skin diseases. Very healing for oozing acne and rashes resulting from poison oak, ivy, sumac, or general contact dermatitis.
Contraindication: Do not use during pregnancy or if you suffer from high blood pressure or epilepsy.

FLORAL WATERS

Floral waters, or aromatic hydrosols, are a pure, natural by-product of the essential oil distillation process. These fragrant waters are saturated with the water-soluble compounds present in the plants and are gentle enough to use when an essential oil would be too strong or would be irritating to a particular skin type or condition.

Hydrosols make wonderful toners, splashes, and sprays that are soothing, hydrating, lightly moisturizing, and mildly antiseptic. Additionally, floral waters can replace distilled plain water in a cream or lotion recipe to increase the therapeutic value and fragrance. They can be purchased in better health food stores and herb shops or from the mail-order companies listed in the resource section.

CHAMOMILE, GERMAN (*MATRICARIA RECUTITA*)
Cosmetic Properties and Uses: Soothing and balancing, good for all skin types, especially sensitive, irritated, and couperose. Powerful anti-inflammatory with a haunting floral, intoxicating, relaxing fragrance.

LAVENDER (*LAVANDULA* SPP.)
Cosmetic Properties and Uses: This classic water has a clean, floral fragrance. Its gentle antiseptic, calming, and healing qualities bring relief to skin irritations and sunburn. An ideal toner for normal or dry skin.

NEROLI or ORANGE BLOSSOM (*CITRUS AURANTIUM*)
Cosmetic Properties and Uses: Sweet, orange/floral fragrance from the flowers of the bitter orange. Acts as a mild, refreshing astringent. Beneficial to acneic, irritated, oily, and sensitive skin.

ROSE OTTO (*ROSA DAMASCENA*)
Cosmetic Properties and Uses: Wonderfully rich, romantic, old-fashioned floral fragrance. Balancing, calming, and mildly astringent. Helps revive tired, devitalized skin and eyes; gentle enough to be used directly on the eyes.

FRUITS

The following is a list of fruits to use in natural skin care recipes. These fruits contain fruit acids, also called alpha-hydroxy acids (AHAs) or beta-hydroxy agents (BHAs), that are extremely good for the skin when applied externally. AHAs dissolve the bond that holds dead skin cells together and increases hydration while BHAs naturally dissolve dry, flaky surface skin and stimulate cell renewal. All skin types from oily to very dry can benefit from these remarkably effective and inexpensive fruit acids.

When purchasing, try to find organically grown fruit. *Note:* For maximum skin rejuvenation, all fruits should be used in their raw state.

APPLE (AHA)
Parts Used: Pulp, freshly pressed juice
Cosmetic Properties and Uses: Contains malic acid. Acts as a mild astringent. Soothing for sensitive and acneic skin. Mixed with white cosmetic clay, makes a gentle, exfoliating mask.

BANANA (AHA)
Parts Used: Pulp
Cosmetic Properties and Uses: Nourishing and moisturizing. Extremely gentle. Recommended for normal and dry skin. Can be used straight as a mask or blended with white cosmetic clay for added exfoliation and tightening.

BLACKBERRY AND RASPBERRY (AHA)
Parts Used: Freshly pressed, strained juice
Cosmetic Properties and Uses: Contains lactic acid. Can be applied with a cotton ball directly to all but the most sensitive or sunburned skin as an exfoliating tonic and then rinsed off. Moderately astringent.

CITRUS FRUITS — GRAPEFRUIT, LEMON, LIME, ORANGE, TANGERINE (AHA)
Parts Used: Freshly pressed juice, rind (zest)
Cosmetic Properties and Uses: Contains citric acid. Astringent and fragrant. Good for oily and normal skin. Juice and zest can be added to toners, spritzers, masks, and lotions.

Contraindication: Not recommended for use on sensitive or inflamed skin.

GRAPE (AHA)
Parts Used: Freshly pressed juice
Cosmetic Properties and Uses: Contains tartaric acid. Apply juice to face with cotton ball to help improve skin texture, rinse. Safe for all skin types.

PAPAYA (BHA)
Parts Used: Pulp
Cosmetic Properties and Uses: Contains the enzyme papain. Applied as a wet mask, helps even out skin tone and soften skin. Especially useful for a fading tan or dry, flaky, rough skin.
Contraindication: May be irritating to sensitive, sunburned, or inflamed skin.

PINEAPPLE (BHA)
Parts Used: Freshly pressed juice
Cosmetic Properties and Uses: Contains the enzyme bromelain. Will dissolve dead, dry skin cells resulting in smoother skin.
Contraindication: May be irritating to sensitive, sunburned, or inflamed skin.

STRAWBERRY (AHA)
Parts Used: Pulp
Cosmetic Properties and Uses: Acts as a gentle astringent. Safe for all skin types. Pulp may be thickened with white cosmetic clay and applied as an exfoliating mask.

GRAINS, NUTS, AND SEEDS

I always have a generous supply of the following four "skin foods" in my kitchen. They are staples for the kitchen cosmetologist. All ingredients should be organically grown, if possible, and used in raw form. To ensure freshness, nuts and seeds should be kept in the freezer. Oatmeal can be stored in a cool, dry cabinet.

MAKING GRAIN, SEED, AND NUT MEALS

Almond Meal

To make ½ cup (125 ml) almond meal, grind (in 10-second pulses) approximately 50 large, raw almonds in a blender, coffee grinder, or food processor until the consistency is that of finely grated Parmesan cheese. Due to their high fat content, it's very easy to overblend almonds and end up with almond butter, especially if you use a small grinder that generates lots of heat. This is actually not a bad thing, as it is quite tasty and can be used just like peanut butter, but it's not the result you're after!

Flaxseed Meal

To make ½ cup (125 ml) flaxseed meal, blend a heaping ½ cup (125 ml) seeds in a blender, coffee grinder, or food processor until the consistency is that of coarse whole wheat flour.

Ground Oatmeal

To make ½ cup (125 ml) ground oatmeal, blend ¾ to 1 cup (180 to 250 ml) of regular or old-fashioned oats in a blender, coffee grinder, or food processor until the consistency is that of fine flour.

Sunflower Seed Meal

To make ½ cup (125 ml) sunflower seed meal, grind ¾ cup (180 ml) of large seeds (hulled) in a blender, coffee grinder, or food processor until the consistency is that of finely grated Parmesan cheese.

ALMOND

Forms Used: Ground almonds (almond meal)
Cosmetic Properties and Uses: High in skin-loving nutrients and fat. Used as a facial and body scrub base to gently exfoliate rough, dry skin.

FLAXSEED

Forms Used: Ground seeds (flaxseed meal) or cracked seeds
Cosmetic Properties and Uses: When water is added to the whole, cracked seeds or meal, the resulting emollient gel can be strained and massaged into the skin to soothe, nourish, and help heal minor irritations, acne, and sunburn.

OATMEAL

Forms Used: Ground oatmeal

Cosmetic Properties and Uses: Added to bath water, oatmeal relieves itchy, rashy skin and allergic reactions from poison ivy, oak, and sumac or insect bites. Ground oatmeal can also be used as a mask base for all skin types and as a gentle facial scrub for sensitive or couperose skin.

SUNFLOWER

Forms Used: Ground seeds (sunflower seed meal)

Cosmetic Properties and Uses: Very rich in fatty acids, emollients, and beneficial nutrients. Meal makes a gentle, moisturizing scrub and mask base for normal-to-dry skin.

HERBS, SPICES, AND FLOWERS

Herbs have been used for thousands of years by every culture for their medicinal, fragrant, and skin-pampering qualities. The following are my favorite herbs for skin care. They are easily found in most health food stores, herb shops, or through mail-order suppliers (see Resources). Try to purchase organically grown herbs if possible, or grow your own. Fresh is always best!

ALOE VERA *(ALOE VERA)*

Parts Used: Gel or juice from the leaves

Cosmetic Properties and Uses: The gel and juice helps heal all types of burns, insect bites, and rashes. Slightly astringent and very soothing. Terrific when mixed with a drop or two of lavender essential oil and sprayed on sunburned skin.

GEL OR JUICE?

Aloe vera gel can be lumpy at times. If you're making a preparation to be spritzed on your face or body, you'll probably prefer to work with aloe vera juice. You can either purchase the juice or make it yourself at home: Mix 1/4 cup (60 ml) of the gel with 1 tablespoon (15 ml) distilled water and blend for 15 seconds.

CALENDULA *(CALENDULA OFFICINALIS)*
Common Name: Pot marigold
Parts Used: Flower petals
Cosmetic Properties and Uses: Contains antifungal, anti-inflamitory, antiseptic, and antibacterial properties. As an infused oil, calendula is healing to cuts, bruises, rashes, and irritated skin when combined with spike lavender, tea tree, German chamomile, or thyme essential oil.

CHAMOMILE, GERMAN *(MATRICARIA RECUTITA)*
Common Names: Blue chamomile, wild chamomile
Parts Used: Flowering tops
Cosmetic Properties and Uses: Cooled tea is a good anti-inflammatory treatment for pimples and acne, and the dried, ground flowers are a good addition to gentle facial scrubs. The whole, fresh flowers can be added to bath water for a relaxing, fragrant, skin-pampering way to end your day.

CINNAMON *(CINNAMOMUM AROMATICUM)*
Common Name: Cassia
Parts Used: Powdered inner bark
Cosmetic Properties and Uses: Mildly astringent, antiseptic, and fragrant. In combination with powdered, dried chamomile flowers, white cosmetic clay, and ground oatmeal, makes a gentle exfoliating scrub or mask.

COMFREY *(SYMPHYTUM OFFICINALE)*
Parts Used: Leaves, root
Cosmetic Properties and Uses: High in minerals, protein, and allantoin. Mildly astringent, emollient, mucilaginous. Tea made from chopped root is healing, skin-nurturing, and speeds cell renewal. A compress can be applied to cuts, burns, eczema, and psoriasis to bring relief to inflammation, swelling, and irritation.

ELDERFLOWER *(SAMBUCUS CANADENSIS)*
Parts Used: Flowers
Cosmetic Properties and Uses: The flowers make a soothing wash for both eye and skin irritations. Good for all skin types.

EYEBRIGHT *(EUPHRASIA ROSTKOVIANA)*

Parts Used: Flowers, stems, and leaves

Cosmetic Properties and Uses: The entire plant is used to make an infusion that soothes irritated, strained eyes. Mildly astringent, antiseptic, and anti-inflammatory.

FENNEL *(FOENICULUM VULGARE)*

Parts Used: Seeds

Cosmetic Properties and Uses: The fragrant, licorice-scented seeds, when added to boiling water, make a deep cleansing facial steam that is especially good for normal-to-dry and wrinkled skin. The tea can be used as a healing tonic for chapped skin.

LAVENDER (*LAVANDULA* SPP.)

Parts Used: Flowers, leaves

Cosmetic Properties and Uses: Can be used as an infusion as a soothing facial wash for all skin types, especially irritated and acneic skin. Ground, dried flowers can be combined with ground oatmeal and used as a calming, gentle facial scrub and mask for even the most sensitive skins.

LEMON BALM *(MELISSA OFFICINALIS)*

Parts Used: Leaves, stems

Cosmetic Properties and Uses: Refreshing lemony fragrance and flavor. The tea is an excellent addition to light lotions and creams to help heal and cleanse skin affected by pimples, acne, insect bites, and rashes. Lemon balm infusion has antiviral properties, which is good for your irritated skin, harmful for pesky bacteria. Combined with vinegar, this herb makes a lovely facial rinse that can be used to balance your skin's pH after cleansing.

LEMONGRASS *(CYMBOPOGON CITRATUS)*

Parts Used: Leaf blades

Cosmetic Properties and Uses: Has a refreshing, lemony fragrance. As a tea, makes an excellent antiseptic for oily skin. Acts as an astringent cleansing agent in facials, steams, and toners.

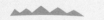

HERB STORAGE TIP

Dried herbs should be stored in dark-colored glass jars, tins, or zip-seal plastic bags, in a dark, cool, dry place. A good-quality herb will keep for up to one year.

HOW TO MAKE AN HERBAL INFUSION

Herbal infusions, teas, or waters are frequently used as an ingredient in splashes, tonics, lotions, creams, and bath additives. To make, pour 1 cup (250 ml) of boiling water over 1 teaspoon (5 ml) dried herb or 2 teaspoons (10 ml) fresh herb. Cover, steep 5 to 10 minutes, and strain. Cool and use as directed.

LICORICE *(GLYCYRRHIZA GLABRA)*

Parts Used: Roots

Cosmetic Properties and Uses: Helps reduce skin inflammation resulting from allergies or rashes. Especially good used in acne treatments and poison plant rashes. Soothing and healing.

MARSH MALLOW *(ALTHAEA OFFICINALIS)*

Parts Used: Roots

Cosmetic Properties and Uses: The Greek word *althaea* means "to heal." Roots contain a soothing mucilage and when steeped in simmering water produce a "healing goo" that is quite beneficial for weather-beaten, chapped, or sun-damaged skin. An excellent anti-inflammatory when applied to acneic skin.

PEPPERMINT *(MENTHA X PIPERITA)*

Parts Used: Leaves, stems

Cosmetic Properties and Uses: Stimulating, refreshing, antiseptic, fragrant, and antiviral. Peppermint vinegar balances the skin's pH after cleansing. Peppermint infusion is cooling to hot, sweaty "summer skin" and has a mild, astringent quality that helps to remove excess oil.

RED CLOVER *(TRIFOLIUM PRATENSE)*

Parts Used: Flowers

Cosmetic Properties and Uses: Often considered a weed, the reddish pink blossoms of this plant are used as an anti-inflammatory, calming, and cleansing ingredient in products for normal-to-dry skin. They're a wonderful addition in facial steam blends for dry, irritated skin.

ROSE (*ROSA* SPP.)

Parts Used: Petals

Cosmetic Properties and Uses: I use the dried, ground petals mixed with white cosmetic clay and ground oatmeal to make a gentle facial exfoliant and mask that can be used by all skin types.

ROSEMARY *(ROSMARINUS OFFICINALIS)*

Parts Used: Leaves

Cosmetic Properties and Uses: An infusion made from the aromatic and antiseptic leaves can be used by all skin types as a facial or body splash, or added to lotions and cream recipes in place of distilled water. Also beneficial in facial steams to help cleanse the pores.

SAGE *(SALVIA OFFICINALIS)*

Parts Used: Leaves, flowers

Cosmetic Properties and Uses: A strongly fragrant infusion made from the astringent and antiseptic leaves is an effective cleanser for normal-to-oily skin. A cup of sage vinegar added to your bath will help relieve itchiness caused by heat rash or poison ivy, oak, or sumac.

THYME *(THYMUS VULGARIS)*

Parts Used: Leaves

Cosmetic Properties and Uses: Disinfectant and antiseptic. Thyme infusion is a good wash for cuts, scrapes, ulcers, and acne. Recommended for normal-to-oily skin. Try to grow a patch in your garden so that you can make fresh thyme vinegar to freshen your skin and also to put in your salad dressing — yum!

YARROW (*ACHILLEA MILLEFOLIUM*)

Parts Used: Leaves, flowers

Cosmetic Properties and Uses: Very strong astringent. A poultice of the crushed, fresh leaves applied to cuts arrests bleeding. A flower infusion can be used to treat eczema and acne.

HOW TO DO A PATCH TEST WITH HERBS

In a small bowl, combine 1/2 teaspoon (2.5 ml) fresh or dried chopped herb in question with 1 teaspoon (5 ml) or so boiling water. Let the herb absorb the water for a few minutes. Apply a dab of the herb to the inside of your upper arm or wrist and cover with an adhesive strip. Leave in place 12 to 24 hours. If no irritation develops, the herb is generally safe to use.

ETHICAL WILDCRAFTING

Ethical wildcrafting, simply put, is the act of harvesting your herbs fresh from the wild and taking care that you don't over-harvest the area. This means that after harvesting there is enough healthy, growing herb remaining on site to continue to spread and repopulate the surrounding environment.

United Plant Savers (see Resources) is an organization that is dedicated to replanting endangered and threatened medicinal plants. Here is an excerpt from their brochure regarding wild-crafting.

◆ Always wildcraft with thoughts of beauty. Put beauty into your work. Ask yourself, "How much more beautiful will this plant community be when I am finished gathering?"

◆ Think first about the plant community and how many plants it can manage without, not how many plants you need in order to make products or profits.

◆ Treat the native plant complexes like the fine perennial gardens that they are.

◆ Do not upset in any manner undisturbed native soil — it is rare and precious.

◆ Take only as many plants as you can reasonably use; strive for zero waste.

◆ Replant the areas you are harvesting from. Scatter seeds, replace crowns and plant roots. Leave plenty of mature and seed-producing plants to reproduce.

◆ Start a replanting project in your area to help reestablish endangered and threatened species.

◆ Know the endangered plant species in your bio-region.

CLAY, SALT, THICKENERS, AND MISCELLANEOUS INGREDIENTS

This section outlines what I call "active ingredients," because they act as emulsifiers and binders, thickeners, humectants, preservatives, and pH balancers. These ingredients can be purchased through better health food and grocery stores, herb shops, and mail-order suppliers (see Resources).

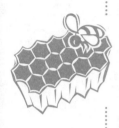

BEESWAX
Form Used: Pure, unrefined, filtered or unfiltered beeswax
Cosmetic Properties and Uses: A thickener for making lip balms, salves, creams, and lotions. Purchase fresh from an apiary, if possible.

BORAX
Form Used: Crystalline powdered mineral salt
Cosmetic Properties and Uses: Can be bought in the laundry aisle of grocery stores. Acts as a binder and texturizer and, when combined with beeswax, oil, and water, makes a stable emulsion. Also acts as a whitener, mild antiseptic, and natural preservative.

CLAY, FRENCH GREEN
Form Used: Dried powder
Cosmetic Properties and Uses: A sage-green, highly mineralized clay, it's especially good for oily skin and for healing conditions that need drawing, astringency, sloughing, or circulation stimulation, such as acne, eczema, psoriasis, and devitalized, wrinkled skin.

CLAY, WHITE COSMETIC
Form Used: Dried powder
Cosmetic Properties and Uses: Preferred in facial care products for sensitive or normal-to-dry skin because of its gentleness. I use it when making masks and scrubs. Draws impurities from your skin, exfoliates, and remineralizes your complexion.

COCOA BUTTER
Form Used: Fatty cocoa wax or butter
Cosmetic Properties and Uses: Acts as a soothing emollient to sunburned and dry skin. Use in lip balms, creams, and lotions to soften the skin and thicken the product. Hardens in cold weather, but melts when applied to the skin.

GLYCERIN, VEGETABLE
Form Used: Clear, sweet thick liquid
Cosmetic Properties and Uses: Acts as a humectant, which means it draws moisture from the air to your skin. Use in lotions and creams for dry skin. Makes lip balms taste super sweet!

GRAPEFRUIT SEED EXTRACT
Common Names: Grapefruit extract, citrus seed extract, citrus extract
Form Used: Concentrated liquid extract
Cosmetic Properties and Uses: Used mainly as an astringent preservative and antimicrobial in the cosmetic industry. I add it to facial and body splashes, creams, and lotions to extend the shelf life of the product.

LANOLIN, ANHYDROUS
Form Used: Fat or wax from sheep's wool
Cosmetic Properties and Uses: An emollient that holds water on the skin. It absorbs water and is a terrific emulsifier for creams and lotions.
Contraindication: May be a potential allergen — do a patch test first (as described on page 9).

SEA SALT
Form Used: Granular sea salt
Cosmetic Properties and Uses: Rich in minerals. Aids in healing oozing, itchy, rashy, inflamed skin. When added to bath water, sea salt can benefit skin afflicted with acne, eczema, psoriasis, poison plant rash, and other irritations.
Contraindication: Limit salt baths to 2 to 3 times per week as this mineral can be drying to the skin. Always follow a salt bath with an application of a good moisturizer.

VINEGAR, RAW APPLE CIDER
Form Used: Diluted vinegar

Cosmetic Properties and Uses: Softens and relieves itchy skin if added to bath water. I use it as a base for making herbal splashes and toners for all skin types. The natural fruit acids in vinegar act as a gentle exfoliant, leaving skin smooth and glowing. Restores normal pH to skin after cleansing.

Contraindication: May irritate sensitive or sunburned skin.

VITAMIN E (D-ALPHA TOCOPHEROL)
Form Used: Liquid capsule form

Cosmetic Properties and Uses: Acts as a natural preservative and antioxidant when added to creams, lotions, and base oils. Helps prevent rancidity. Reported to soften and gradually fade scar tissue. Fabulous relief for chapped lips and ragged cuticles.

WATER, DISTILLED
Form Used: Steam-distilled water

Cosmetic Properties and Uses: Used in making all cosmetic

WHAT DOES PH MEAN?

The pH (potential hydrogen) of a liquid refers to its degree of acidity or alkalinity. The pH scale goes from 0 to 14, with the neutral point being 7. Anything below a 7 on the pH scale is regarded as acid, and anything above 7 is considered alkaline. The lower the pH, the greater the degree of acidity; the higher the pH, the greater the degree of alkalinity. The pH of normal, healthy skin ranges from 4.5 to 6 and is most often given as 5.5.

Most soaps and shampoos have a pH value between 8 and 11, quite alkaline, while most toners and facial splashes have a pH value of between 4.5 and 6, more on the "skin-loving" acid side.

Your skin maintains its proper pH level by forming an acid mantle on its surface with the combined secretions of your sweat and oil glands. Using a toner after cleansing will keep your skin at its proper pH level, helping to prevent bacterial penetration (which can occur when skin is too acidic) and flaking and scaling due to moisture loss (which can occur when skin is too alkaline). Diluted herbal vinegars are ideal for restoring normal skin pH.

products that call for water or herb infusions. Will discourage premature mold growth in your cosmetics, which may occur if you use plain tap water.

WITCH HAZEL
Form Used: Liquid, water- and alcohol-based extract of witch hazel herb
Cosmetic Properties and Uses: Mild astringent. The ideal cleanser for minor cuts, scratches, and pimples. I use it as a facial splash base for normal-to-oily skin. The drugstore variety is fine.

TOOLS, CONTAINERS, AND SUPPLIES

Whether preparing skin care products or dinner for six, the same sanitary precautions apply. Always wash your hands, pots, pans, knives, spoons, whisks, spatulas, blender, cutting board, and every other tool you'll be using in very hot, soapy water. You want to minimize the potential for harmful bacterial growth.

Containers for your final products should be sterilized. There are a few different methods you can use:

- Run them through the dishwasher.
- Soak them in very hot, soapy water combined with a bit of bleach (approximately 1 tablespoon [5 ml] for every gallon [4 l] of water) for approximately 15 minutes; then give them a good scrub to wash off the bleach.
- If you have glass containers, immerse them in boiling water for 1 minute.

Equipment

Preparing skin care products requires only common, everyday kitchen equipment. Here's a list of what you will need:

BLENDER
Useful for making lotions or creams in quantities of 1 cup or more. A blender can also be used to grind oatmeal, nuts, seeds, and herbs, but a nut/seed or coffee grinder does a better job.

BOWLS

Use glass, plastic, stainless-steel, enamel, or ceramic bowls. Make sure they're easy to clean and comfortable to hold. You'll need a variety of sizes, from the smallest ramekin for mixing single-serving facial scrubs to a large mixing bowl for facial steams.

COFFEE GRINDER

This kitchen gadget gets more use than any other piece of equipment I own. It's basically the same as a nut/seed grinder. I grind oatmeal, almonds, seeds, and flowers into powders for facial and body scrubs and masks. I use separate grinders for my cosmetics and my coffee — coffee beans leave a lingering flavor and aroma in the grinder that will permeate your natural skin care ingredients, tainting your products.

CUTTING BOARD

Used for slicing and dicing miscellaneous items. I keep a separate cutting board for processing any meat products. Always keep your boards extremely clean by washing them in hot, soapy water with a bit of bleach added for extra disinfecting.

DOUBLE BOILER

This piece of equipment is used to melt wax, cocoa butter, or coconut oil, and to warm oils when making various creams, lotions, and lip balms. The advantage of a double boiler is that it produces a gentle, even heat, making it impossible to scorch

Most of the equipment and utensils you'll need for making your own herbal preparations can already be found right in your kitchen.

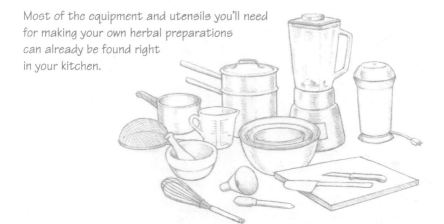

your ingredients if you suddenly get called away from the kitchen. If you don't have a double boiler, a stainless-steel pan (or pans) to melt and warm ingredients is fine if placed over the lowest setting on the stove and its contents stirred occasionally.

EYEDROPPERS

Glass eyedroppers are useful for measuring essential oils by the drop. I try to have a separate one for each oil. Sterilize your droppers every so often by pouring rubbing alcohol through them. Purchase droppers from mail-order herb supply stores, craft stores, bottle companies, or drugstores.

FUNNELS

A small funnel (plastic or stainless-steel) comes in handy when pouring liquid recipes into narrow-necked storage bottles. Funnels come in various sizes and are available in most hardware and grocery stores.

MEASURING CUPS AND SPOONS

Preparing creams and lotions frequently requires exacting measurements; that's where these come in handy.

MORTAR AND PESTLE

Usually available in three sizes, approximately 3, 4½, or 6 inches (7.5, 11.3, or 15 cm) in diameter, and made from marble, polished granite, colored and sandblasted glass, or wood. I prefer the larger stone variety because of its heft. It is perfect for crushing dried seeds, herbs, and spices; for mashing fresh herbs, flowers, and blackberries or raspberries to extract their juices; and to make spreadable pulp pastes from fruits such as pineapple, papaya, and strawberries. These are sold in better hardware stores, kitchen supply stores, some herb shops and health food stores, or through mail-order suppliers.

POTS AND PANS

Stainless-steel, enamel, or glass only, please. Best to have a variety of sizes, including a 1-pint (500 ml) saucepan and 1-, 2-, and 3-quart (1-, 2-, and 3-liter) pots. I use all sizes for melting oils and beeswax as well as for making herb tea and extracting mucilaginous substances from herb roots.

PARING KNIVES

I always have several sharp blades at my disposal. I cut beeswax with a paring knife instead of using a cheese grater. It's easier on my knuckles! Be sure to keep your knives sharp. My good friend Hervé works as a produce clerk at the local grocery store and is constantly opening boxes and crates using a big, sharp knife. He informs me that most knife injuries are the result of using a dull knife, not a sharp one. "A dull knife," he says, "requires more pressure on your part to cut a piece of fruit, an herb stem, or a vegetable, thus increasing the likelihood of slipping and cutting your finger instead."

SPATULA

A spatula is better than a spoon for scooping out creams and lotions from any type of container. I recommend keeping a variety of sizes on hand.

STRAINER

I use a woven bamboo or standard mesh strainer for straining liquids that contain large herb matter. For straining finely ground materials, I line either of these strainers with cheesecloth or a nylon stocking.

WHISK

A small wire whisk is great for blending and whipping a small quantity of lotion, cream, salve, or lip balm.

FOR SAFETY'S SAKE

Though most of the ingredients in the skin care recipes included in this book are safe to consume, some, essential oils for example, can be quite harmful. Please label each product you make and store away from pets and children.

Containers

Obviously, if you make an herbal product you have to store it in something, and the more attractive the container, the better. Cosmetic companies know that packaging sells — frequently the pretty package costs more to produce than the ingredients inside! What I'm trying to say is this: If you store your fresh rosemary face cream in an old mustard jar, you won't be as apt to use it as you would if you stored it in an aesthetically pleasing jar.

Discount import/export shops and flea markets often carry scads of bottles and jars for the herbal crafter at really great prices. Herb shops and health food stores, though, can be rather expensive places to purchase individual bottles. Antiques shops often sell really unique containers if you're looking for something special. I generally purchase my containers by the case from mail-order bottle companies (see Resources). As always, buying in bulk saves money.

Don't forget to label your skin care creations. A simple custom label looks professional and your friends will want to purchase some of your wares for gift-giving. Ever thought of starting an herbal craft business? If so, check out the following informative books: *Growing Your Herb Business* and *Creating an Herbal Bodycare Business.*

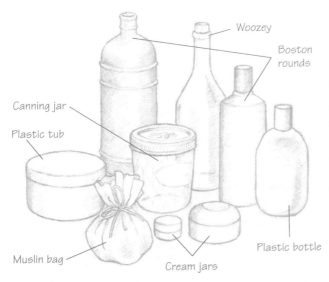

Woozey

Boston rounds

Canning jar

Plastic tub

Muslin bag

Cream jars

Plastic bottle

There are a multitude of containers to choose from for storing your preparations and formulas, including but not limited to the ones shown here.

BOSTON ROUNDS

A Boston round is a glass container perfect for spritzers, lotions, and oils. They come in myriad colors: amber, clear, green, and cobalt blue, and in sizes from ½ ounce to 16 ounces (15 to 450 g). Darker colored glass will protect your herbal products from light damage. They can be topped with a simple plastic cap, lotion pump, glass dropper, or mister.

CANNING JARS

From half-pint to gallon (250 ml to 4 liter) size, these are suitable for storing dried herbs. The half-pint size is perfect for packaging your wares to give to friends. Slap on your custom label and *voilà!* you've got a beautiful present!

CREAM JARS

Available in different sizes from ¼- to 4-ounce (7- to 115-g) jars. Perfect for creams, lip balms, and healing salves. Available in glass or plastic.

MUSLIN BAGS

Available in a variety of sizes and are useful for making bath bags or large quantities of herbal tea. They are easy to make or can be purchased from craft stores or mail-order suppliers.

PLASTIC BOTTLES

From 2 ounces to 16 ounces (60 to 500 ml), and larger. These can be used for the same products as Boston rounds, except they do not protect the herbal contents from light damage. Better to use if you travel or frequently have children in your bathroom.

PLASTIC TUBS

These are plastic food storage containers with a good-fitting, airtight lid, available in all grocery stores. I use them to store dry facial and body scrubs and mask blends.

WOOZEYS

Designed mainly for culinary use as wine and vinegar bottles, these narrow-necked bottles are super for storing facial and body splashes, floral waters, and bath oils.

DRYING YOUR OWN HERBS

You may be surprised by how easy it is to dry many of the herbs from your garden. No matter which technique you choose, it is best to dry your herbs as soon as they are picked so that none of their beneficial properties are lost. Here are some other points to keep in mind:

- ◆ Harvest herbs as soon as they come into bloom.
- ◆ Using a sharp knife, gather herbs in the early to mid-morning after any evening dew has had a chance to dry but before the sun becomes too hot.
- ◆ Harvest herbs that are free of insects, disease, and have not been treated with pesticides. Herbs should be relatively dirt-free but if they are dusty you can quickly rinse them in cool water and immediately pat dry with a paper towel. Be sure to pat gently as the leaves will bruise easily.
- ◆ Avoid overdrying as it can diminish the valuable properties of the herb.
- ◆ Dried herbs should be stored in a cool, moisture-free place away from direct sunlight.

Drying by Hanging

To dry your herbs by hanging, simply gather five stems of a single herb together in a bundle. Secure the stems together using a string, rubber bands, or clothes pins. Bundles should be hung upside down in a well-ventilated, dimly lit area. The ideal temperature for drying is between 65°F (20°C) and 80°F (25°C). Leave plenty of room between bundles to ensure good air circulation and to keep scents from mingling. As many herbs look similar when dried, you may find it helpful to label your bundles.

Herbs can take anywhere from four days to three weeks to dry. Leaves should be brittle but not so dry as to easily shatter. Flower petals should feel dry and crisp.

Drying on Screens

Many herbs can also be successfully dried on wire screens or tightly stretched netting. The open mesh of the screen or net allows air to flow freely around the herb and quickly evaporate the plants' moisture.

To prepare herbs for screen drying, separate the leaves and flower petals from the stem and spread in a single layer over the screen. Leave enough space between leaves and petals to allow for good air circulation. Drying times will vary between four days and three weeks.

RESOURCES

Bottles and Jars

Burch Bottle and Packaging
430 Hudson River Road
Waterford, NY 12188
(800) 903-2830
www.burchbottle.com

E.D. Luce Prescription
  Packaging
1600 East 29th Street
Signal Hill, CA 90806
(562) 997-9777
www.essentialsupplies.com

SKS Bottle and Packaging
3 Knabner Road
Mechanicville, NY 12118
(518) 899-7488
www.sks-bottle.com

Sunburst Bottle Company
5710 Auburn Boulevard #7
Sacramento, CA 95841
(916) 348-5576
www.sunburstbottle.com

Herb and Natural Product Suppliers

Aroma Vera
5310 Beethoven Street
Los Angeles, CA 90016
(800) 669-9514 ext. 4705
www.aromavera.com

Aromaland
1326 Rufina Circle
Sante Fe, NM 87507
(800) 933-5267
www.aromaland.com

Atlantic Spice Company
P.O. Box 205
North Truro, MA 02652
(800) 316-7965
www.altanticspice.com

Aura Cacia
P.O. Box 311
Norway, IA 52318
(800) 437-3301
www.frontiercoop.com

Avena Botanicals
219 Mill Street
Rockport, ME 04856
(207) 594-0694

Boericke & Tafel
2381 Circadian Way
Santa Rosa, CA 95407
(707) 571-8202

Brushy Mountain Bee Farm
610 Bethany Church Road
Moravian Falls, NC 28654
(800) BEESWAX

Dry Creek Herb Farm
14245 Edgehill Lane
Auburn, CA 95603
(530) 888-0889
www.drycreekherb farm.com

The Essential Oil Company
1719 SE Umatilla Street
Portland, OR 97202
(800) 729-5912
www.essentialoil.com

Fleur Aromatherapy
Langston Priory Mews
Kingham, Oxon
OX7 6UP, UK
+44 (0) 1608 659 909,
www.fleur.co.uk/front
  page.html

Frontier Co-op Herbs
P.O. Box 299
Norway, IA 52318
(800) 669-3275
www.frontiercoop.com

Janca's
456 East Juanita #7
Mesa, AZ 85204
(480) 497-9494
www.jancas.com

Jean's Greens
119 Sulphur Springs Road
Norway, NY 13416
(888) 845-8327
www.jeansgreens.com

Lavender Lane
7337 #1 Roseville Road
Sacramento, CA 95842
(888) 593-4400
www.lavenderlane.com

Liberty Natural Products
8120 SE Stark Street
Portland, OR 97215
(800) 289-8427
www.libertynatural.com

Motherlove Herbal
  Company
P.O. Box 101
LaPorte, CO 80535
(970) 493-2892
www.motherlove.com

Mountain Rose Herbs
85472 Dilley Lane
Eugene, OR 97405
(800) 879-3337
www.mountainrose
  herbs.com

Norfolk Lavender
777 New Durham Road
Edison, NJ 08817
(800) 886-0050
www.norfolklavender.com

Pacific Botanicals
4350 Fish Hatchery Road
Grants Pass, OR 97527
(541) 479-7777
www.pacificbotanicals.com

Pacific Institute of
  Aromatherapy
P.O. Box 6723
San Rafael, CA 94903
(415) 479-9120
www.pacificinstituteof
  aromatherapy.com

Penn Herb Company
10601 Decatur Road
Philadelphia, PA 19154
(800) 523-9971
www.pacificbotanicals.com

Sage Woman Herbs
406 S. 8th Street
Colorado Springs, CO
    80905
(800) 350-3911
www.sagewomanherbs.com

September's Sun Herbal
    Soap and Skin Care
    Company
Stephanie Tourles, Owner
P.O. Box 772
W. Hyanisport, MA 02672
(508) 862-9955

Shirley Price
    Aromatherapy Ltd.
Essentia House
Upper Bond Street
Hincley, Leicestershire
LE10 1RS, UK
+44 (0) 14 5561 5466
www.shirleyprice.com

Vermont Country Store
P.O. Box 3000
Manchester Center, VT
    05255
(802) 362-2400
www.vermontcountry
    store.com

**Education and
Associations**

The American Association
    for Health Freedom
P.O. Box 458
Great Falls, VA 22066
(800) 230-2762
www.healthfreedom.net

American Association of
    Naturopathic Physicians
8201 Greensboro Drive,
    Suite 300
McLean, VA 22102
(877) 969-2267
www.naturopathic.org

American Botanical
    Council
P.O. Box 144345
Austin, TX 78714
(512) 926-4900

American Herb Assoc.
P.O. Box 1673
Nevada City, CA 95959
(530) 265-9552

American Herbal Products
    Association
8484 Georgia Ave., Ste. 370
Silver Spring, MD 20910
(301) 588-1174

American Herbalist's Guild
1931 Gaddis Road
Canton, GA 30115
(770) 751-6021
www.americanherbalist.com

Bio-Dynamic Farming and
    Gardening Association
P.O. Box 29135
San Francisco, CA 94129
(888) 516-7797
www.biodynamics.com

Citizens for Health
5 Thomas Circle NW,
    Suite 500
Washington, DC 20005
(202) 483-1652
www.citizens.org

Community Alliance with
    Family Farmers
P.O. Box 363
Davis, CA 95617
(800) 852-3832

Herb Growing and
    Marketing Network
P.O. Box 245
Silver Spring, PA 17575
(717) 393-3295
www.herbnet.com

Herb Research Foundation
1007 Pearl Street Ste. 200
Boulder, CO 80302
(303) 449-2265
www.herbs.org

International Federation
    of Aromatherapists
182 Chiswick High Road
London W4 1PP, UK
+44 (0) 20 8742 2605
www.int-fed-aroma
    therapy.co.uk

International Society of
    Aromatherapists
ISPA House, 82 Ashby Rd.
Hinckley, Leicestershire
LE10 1SN, UK
+44 (0) 14 5563 7987,
www.the-ispa.org

Kerr Center for
    Sustainable Agriculture
P.O. Box 588
Poteau, OK 74953
(918) 647-9123
www.kerrcenter.com

Lady Bird Johnson
    Wildflower Center
4801 LaCrosse Avenue
Austin, TX 78739
(512) 292-4200
www.wildflower.org

Northeast Herbal Assoc.
P.O. Box 103
Manchaug, MA 01526
www.northeastherbal.org

United Plant Savers
P.O. Box 98
East Barre, VT 05649
www.plantsavers.org

**Periodicals
and Publications**

Acres USA: A Voice for
    Eco-Agriculture
P.O. Box 91299
Austin, TX 78709
(800) 355-5313
www.acresusa.com

Dandelion Doings
Goosefoot Acres, Inc.
P.O. Box 18016
Cleveland, OH 44118
(216) 932-2145
www.edibleweeds.com

The Herb Companion
Interweave Press, Inc.
243 East Fourth Street
Loveland, CO 80537
(800) 272-2193
www.discoverherbs.com

INDEX

overscrubbing with,
239
skin, 4
Cleansing and Rejuvenat-
ing Oil (recipe), 21
Cocoa butter, 327
Cocoa Butter Lotion for
Face and Body (recipe),
32
Coconut fiber brush, 162
Coconut Palm Oil, 307
Cold feet. *See* Foot prob-
lems and remedies
Cold-pressed oils, 305
Cold sores, 289–291
recipes for, 69, 291
Comfrey *(Symphytum
officinale)*, 321
Comfrey/Calendula Heal-
ing Salve (recipe), 302
Conditioners, hair. *See*
Hair
Constipation, 239, 261
Containers. *See* Storage
Cool Potato Burn Relief
(recipe), 133
Corn pads for feet, 147
Cornmeal and Honey
Scrub (recipe), 16
Corns. *See* Foot problems
and remedies
Cortisone, 274, 283
for hives, 294
for psoriasis, 299
Cosmetics, 248
Couperose, 268–270
Creams and lotions. *See
also* Moisturizers
cleansing, 18–22
Creamy Scrub Cleanser
(recipe), 13
Cuts and scrapes, 270–272
Cymbopogon citratus
(Lemongrass), 313, 322
Cysts. *See* Acne

D

D-alpha Tocopherol (Vita-
min E), 329
Dandruff. *See* Hair
Daucus carota, 309
Deep Pore Cleanser
(recipe), 39

Dehydrated skin. *See* Skin,
dry
Dentifrices. *See* Tooth-
paste
Dermatitis, 272–274, 278
Dermatologist, defined,
245
De-Stressing Foot Bath
(recipe), 177
Diabetes
and cold feet, 197, 198
and effect on nails, 98,
214
and foot treatments,
185, 186, 190, 199,
202–205, 207, 220
Diaper rash
cream for, 34, 271
Diet
and acne, 245
and cellulite, 261, 263
and cold feet, 197, 198
and couperose, 270
and dandruff, 67
and diabetes, 204
and dry, cracked feet,
205
and eczema, 280
and eyes, 284
as factor in skin health,
3
and healthy hands, 79
and hives, 293
and nail health, 92–94,
96–97
and psoriasis, 298
Dr. Mom's Herbal Healing
Cream (recipe), 196
Douches, 73
Drugs, 239
and effect on eyes, 284
and psoriasis, 298
Dry brushing, for skin,
6–7, 263
Dry skin. *See* Skin, dry
Dry Skin Sauna (recipe), 46
Drying herbs, 335

E

EFAs. *See* Essential Fatty
Acids

Eczema, 278–279, *278*
and burdock seed oil,
127
and calendula oil, 304
and effect on nails, 96
foot mask for, 163
and gardening gloves,
81
Egg White Firming Mask
(recipe), 36
Elderflower *(Sambucus
canadensis)*, 321
Elderflower Toner (recipe),
29
Environmentally damaged
skin, 237–238
Equipment and tools
for foot care, 150–153,
151, 154
for making home health
care products, 329–332,
330
Essential fatty acids
(EFAs), 276, 280, 281
Essential oils. *See* Oils,
essential
Esthetician, defined, 245
Eucalyptus *(Eucalyptus
dives)*, 310
Eucalyptus dives (Eucalyptus), 310
Euphrasia rostkoviana
(Eyebright), 322
Evening primrose oil, and
eczema, 281
Everlasting or Immortelle
(Helichrysum italicum),
311
Exercise
as cause of heel spurs,
208
and cellulite, 261, 262,
263
and diabetes, 204
and eczema, 280
as factor in skin health,
3, 241
for feet, 164–171,
165–171, 198
and healthy hands, 79,
88–89, *89*
and hives, 292
and psoriasis, 298